NUTRITION AND DIET RESEARCH PROGRESS

VITAMIN C: NUTRITIONAL ROLE, SUPPLEMENTATION IN PATHOPHYSIOLOGICAL STATES AND SIDE EFFECTS

NUTRITION AND DIET RESEARCH PROGRESS

Additional books in this series can be found on Nova's website under the Series tab.

Additional E-books in this series can be found on Nova's website under the E-books tab.

NUTRITION AND DIET RESEARCH PROGRESS

VITAMIN C: NUTRITIONAL ROLE, SUPPLEMENTATION IN PATHOPHYSIOLOGICAL STATES AND SIDE EFFECTS

RAMÓN RODRIGO
AND
ANDRÉS MIRANDA

Nova Biomedical
Nova Science Publishers, Inc.
New York

For permission to use material from this book please contact us:
Telephone 631-231-7269; Fax 631-231-8175
Web Site: http://www.novapublishers.com

Library of Congress Cataloging-in-Publication Data

Available upon Request
ISBN: 978-1-61728-950-7

Published by Nova Science Publishers, Inc. ✢ New York

Contents

Preface

Vitamin C is a potent water-soluble antioxidant in humans. Although this six-carbon lactone is derived from glucose in most mammalian species, where it is formed mainly in the liver, humans do not possess the enzymes for its synthesis. It is present in various foods, particularly of plant origin, in quantities that are several orders of magnitude higher than those of other vitamins.

At the cell level, vitamin C exerts a protective effect against the oxidation of biomolecules, by many agents such reactive oxygen species produced in both physiological and pathophysiological processes. This protection involves proteins, lipids and DNA.

The growing evidence of the involvement of oxidative stress in the mechanism of non-infectious, chronic and degenerative disorders makes the antioxidant supplementation with vitamin C, an attractive strategy in the prevention and attenuation of progression of these diseases. In the present chapter we are aimed to provide evidence of vitamin C supplementation in the treatment and prevention of important human diseases, such as preeclampsia, hypertension, atherosclerosis, diabetes, among others.

In addition, although this antioxidant vitamin is well tolerated, we include some studies related with its side effects, such as kidney stones formation, diarrhea and indigestion. The underlying mechanisms accounting for these undesirable effects remain to be determined, whereas the prevailing viewpoints consider vitamin C as a safety supplement.

Chapter I

Introduction

It has been known for a long time that the absence of fresh fruits and vegetables in the human diet leads to scurvy – a fatal disease affecting sailors [1] and soldiers [2] in the past. Thus, diet for humans to survive must contain ascorbate. This raises the following questions: which are the most important features of ascorbate, and why does its deficiency have fatal consequences? [3]

In the last decades, attention has been drawn to antioxidant properties of vitamins, such as vitamin C (or L-ascorbic acid; hereafter, 'ascorbic acid' and 'ascorbate' will always refer to 'L-ascorbic acid' and 'L-ascorbate'). Indeed, many of the new insights to mechanisms of disease place oxidative stress as a cornerstone to be addressed. It is in this context that antioxidant vitamin supplementation seems to be a novel strategy to interfere these pathophysiological states.

Many vitamin C nutritional requirements values – both for health and disease - have been proposed because this vitamin C has the particularity of being unable to be synthesized by humans. This recommendations many times lacked an appropriate pharmacokinetic approach, leading to useless practice.

Fortunately, much advance has been made regarding these issues. Biochemical studies have elucidated vitamin C-specific transport mechanisms in humans. Furthermore, at the cellular level, biochemical routes and connections to pathophysiological states have been demonstrated.

Even so, little would we be saying about ascorbate if only to its antioxidant function we would be addressing. The fundamental role for vitamin C in collagen synthesis has been recognized, which historically has been at hand by merely taking into consideration the clinical manifestations of scurvy. Moreover, new properties of the neurotransmission in the brain open a wide new context for investigation on this pleiotropic vitamin's biological functions.

A brief gaze at scurvy is also necessary to bear in mind the function of this vitamin. It is also important due to its appearance in particular populations.

Considering the aforementioned, many clinical publications have focused on this vitamin in order to tackle pathophysiological states. Here we introduce an updated review of the literature on some human epidemiologically relevant diseases or disease-related mechanisms. This further underlies the importance of finding proper strategies to treat disease in an effective, low cost and safe way. All these criteria are certainly fulfilled by ascorbate, which has found to have interesting and promising results on this field. For example, essential hypertensive patients are likely to receive benefit from these supplementations.

The cost/benefit ratio favors Vitamin C use since side effects have not been totally proven. In addition, the features of vitamin C these effects include low frequency, being harmless and dose dependence. Thus, accurate administration seems to be more than enough to address this issue.

Dr. Albert Szent-Györgyi received the 1937 Nobel Prize in Physiology or Medicine, in part for his discovery that hexuronic acid, isolated from adrenal gland, turned out to be vitamin C. Dr. Szent-Györgyi stated in a foreword to a book authored by Irwin Stone entitled "The Healing Factor. Vitamin C Against Disease" [4]:

> "...All the same, I always had the feeling that not enough use was made of it [vitamin C] for supporting human health. The reasons are rather complex. The medical profession itself took a very narrow and very wrong view. Lack of ascorbic acid caused scurvy, so if there was no scurvy there was no lack of ascorbic acid. Nothing could be clearer than this. The only trouble was that scurvy is not a first symptom of a lack but a final collapse, a pre-mortal syndrome and there is a very wide gap between scurvy and full health."

Chapter II

Nutrition

A. Nutritional Requirements

Vitamin C is an essential micronutrient that serves as an antioxidant scavenger of free radicals and as a cofactor in many enzymatic reactions [5].

Ascorbate is found in many fruits and vegetables [6]. Citrus fruits and juices are particularly rich sources of vitamin C but other fruits including cantaloupe and honeydew melons, cherries, kiwi fruits, mangoes, papaya, strawberries, tangelo, tomatoes, and water melon also contain variable amounts of vitamin C. Vegetables such as cabbage, broccoli, Brussels sprouts, bean sprouts, cauliflower, kale, mustard greens, red and green peppers, peas, and potatoes may be more important sources of vitamin C than fruits, given that the vegetable supply often extends for longer periods during the year than does the fruit supply [7].

Indeed, high values for ascorbic acid were obtained for natural orange juice made by fruit squeezing: 30.48 mg/100mL [8]. Thus, 200 to 300 ml of squeezed natural orange juice will provide enough vitamin C for almost any healthy adult.

At present, vitamin C deficiency states are extremely uncommon in humans and one could usually obtain it from consumption of a well-balanced diet [9, 10]. The average body pool of vitamin C is 1.5 g, of which 3%–4% (40 –60 mg) is used daily [11].

Recommended nutrient intakes for vitamin C

The following tables present (Tables 1-3) a summary of the discussed recommended nutrient intakes (RNIs) for vitamin C by group. RNI is the daily intake which meets the nutrient requirements of almost all apparently healthy individuals in an age- and sex-specific population group. The definition of RNI utilized in this chapter is equivalent to that of the recommended dietary allowance (RDA) as used by the Food and Nutrition Board of the United States National Academy of Sciences [12]. For further details on definitions, refer to WHO, 2004 [7].

Table 1. Recommended nutrient intakes (RNIs) for vitamin C, by group

Group	RNI (mg/day)[a]
Infants and children	
0–6 months	25
7–12 months	30[b]
1–3 years	30[b]
4–6 years	30[b]
7–9 years	35[b]
Adolescents	
10–18 years	40[b]
Adults	
19–65 years	45
65+ years	45
Pregnant women	55
Lactating women	70

[a] Amount required to half saturate body tissues with vitamin C in 97.5% of the population. Larger amounts may often be required to ensure adequate absorption of non-haem iron.

[b] Arbitrary values. Data collected from WHO, 2004 [7].

A recent publication [11] highlights the fact that some biochemical functions of vitamin C make it an essential component of parenteral nutrition (PN) and an important therapeutic supplement in other acute conditions. Shocked surgical, trauma, and septic patients have a drastic reduction of circulating plasma ascorbate concentrations. These low concentrations require 3 g/day-doses to restore normal plasma ascorbate concentrations, questioning the recommended PN dose of 100 mg/d. Determination of intravenous requirements is usually based on plasma concentrations, which are altered during the inflammatory response. On the basis of available pharmacokinetic data the 100 mg/d dose for patients receiving home PN and 200 mg/d for stable adult patients receiving PN are adequate, but requirements have been shown to be higher in perioperative, trauma, burn, and critically ill patients, paralleling oxidative stress. One recommendation cannot fit all categories of patients. Large vitamin C supplements may be considered in severe critical illness, major trauma, and burns because of increased requirements resulting from oxidative stress and wound healing.

Table 2. RDA by group

Age	Dose per day		Recommendation
	Men	Women	
0–6 months	40 mg (227 μmol)		AI*
7–12 months	50 mg (256 μmol)		AI*
1–3 years	15 mg (85 μmol)		RDA
4–8 years	25 mg (142 μmol)		RDA
9–13 years	45 mg (256 μmol)	45 mg (256 μmol)	RDA
14–18 years	75 mg (426 μmol)	65 mg (370 μmol)	RDA
19–30 years	90 mg (511 μmol)	75 mg (426 μmol)	RDA
31–50 years	90 mg (511 μmol)	75 mg (426 μmol)	RDA
51–70 years	90 mg (511 μmol)	75 mg (426 μmol)	RDA
>70 years	90 mg (511 μmol)	75 mg (426 μmol)	RDA

*: Adequate intake: value given when sufficient scientific evidence is not available to calculate an estimated average requirement (EAR), from which the RDA is then calculated. Data collected from U.S. Food and Nutrition Board [13].

Table 3. Data collected from U.S. Food and Nutrition Board [13]

Age	Dose per day	
	Pregnancy	Lactation
14–18 years	80 mg (454 μmol)	115 mg (653 μmol)
19–30 years	85 mg (483 μmol)	120 mg (682 μmol)
31–50 years	85 mg (483 μmol)	120 mg (682 μmol)

A positive association between vitamin C consumption and health status has been frequently claimed, but results from intervention studies are inconsistent so far. Low plasma concentrations are reported in patients with diabetes [14] and infections [15] and in smokers [16], but the relative contribution of diet and stress to these situations is uncertain. Epidemiological studies indicate that high vitamin C content diets have been associated with lower cancer risk, especially for cancers of the oral cavity, oesophagus, stomach, colon, and lung [17-20]. However, there appears to be no effect of consumption of vitamin C supplements on the development of colorectal adenoma and stomach cancer [20-22]. Currently there is no consistent evidence from population studies that heart disease, cancers, or cataract development are specifically associated with vitamin C status. This of course does not preclude the possibility that other components in vitamin C-rich fruits and vegetables provide health benefits, but it is not yet possible to isolate such effects from other factors such as lifestyle patterns of people who have a high vitamin C intake.

Early reports in the literature suggested that a minimal intake (i.e., 80 milligrams a day) might not be optimal because low doses could result in degenerative diseases, a compromised immune system and reduced ability to respond to stress [4, 23]. The mega-dose hypothesis popularized by Pauling and Stone, suggested that individuals needed 4 to 20 grams of oral ascorbate per day [4, 23]. They based their hypothesis largely on evolutionary arguments. Most animals synthesize large amounts of ascorbate internally or, less commonly, obtain equivalent gram-level intakes from their diets. Animals also increase their production of vitamin C when they are diseased. Therefore, it was proposed that higher doses provided increased resistance to many, if not all, diseases.

Shortly after Pauling's death, researchers from the National Institute of Health (NIH) published various papers on the pharmacokinetics of oral ascorbate [24-26]. The result led to a widespread assumption that the mega-dose hypothesis was wrong. In fact, it was reported that doses of vitamin C as low as 200 mg per day saturate the body and, therefore, higher doses seem to be unnecessary. This saturation claim was highly influential, becoming a cornerstone of Recommended Dietary Allowance (RDA) [27].

Furthermore, considering the potential side effects, it has been agreed that 1 g of vitamin C appears to be the advisable upper limit of dietary intake per day [7].

B. Chemistry

Vitamin C is a potent water-soluble antioxidant in humans. It is a six-carbon lactone synthesized from glucose in the most mammalian species, mainly in liver, but not in humans [28].

Vitamin C is unique among vitamins for several reasons. It is present in various foods, particularly of plant origin, in quantities (typically 10–100 mg/100 g [29]) that are several orders of magnitude higher than those of other vitamins. This is certainly related to the facts that it is formed from sugars, which are abundant compounds, and that its biochemical synthesis is rather simple.

Another unique aspect of ascorbic acid is that it is a vitamin for only a few vertebrate species, those which have lost the capacity to synthesize it. Early enzymological studies identified L-gulonolactone oxidase (GLO) deficiency as the reason for the inability of some species such as man and guinea pig to synthesize their own vitamin C [30]. GLO, a microsomal enzyme, catalyzes aerobically the conversion of L-gulonolactone to L-ascorbate with production of H_2O_2 [30,31]. Man [32] and guinea pig [33] both have a gene homologous to the rat GLO gene, but they are highly mutated. The inactivation of the GLO gene occurred approximately 40 million years ago [32].

From a structural point of view, ascorbate is also one of the rare compounds containing a hydroxyl group that is so acidic as to be completely dissociated at neutral pH (carbon-3 hydroxyl $pK_a = 4.2$). This is related to the fact that ascorbic acid comprises two conjugated double bonds and that a resonance form can be written for the deprotonated monoanionic form (Figure 1). Resonance forms can also be written for the form of vitamin C that has lost one electron, making the radical semidehydroascorbate (SDA) much more stable, and thus much less reactive, than most other free radicals [34]. It can be detected at 10 nM concentrations in biological fluids by electron paramagnetic resonance spectroscopy [35].

Vitamin C is therefore able to play the role of a free-radical scavenger [36], reacting with highly oxidizing species to replace them by a much less reactive and, moreover, enzymatically recyclable one, SDA. Ascorbate is certainly the most abundant water-soluble compound acting in one-electron reactions, and this is most probably why it plays the role of a cofactor in reactions catalyzed by a number of metal-dependent oxygenases [37].

Vitamin C is very labile, and its loss of vitamin C on boiling milk provides a dramatic example of a cause of infantile scurvy [7].

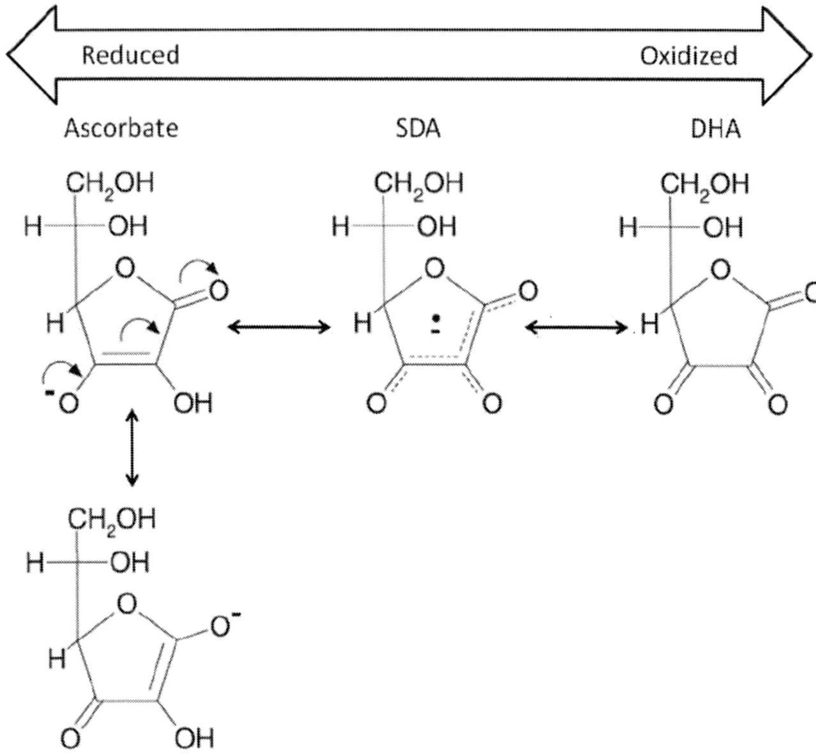

Figure 1. The three redox states of vitamin C (ascorbate, fully reduced form; SDA, monooxidized form; DHA, fully oxidized form), and stabilization of the ascorbate monoanion and SDA by electron delocalization. SDA, semidehydroascorbate; DHA, dehydroascorbate.

C. Pharmacokinetics

After oral intake, for amounts (as much as 300 mg daily) that can be obtained from food, vitamin C plasma concentrations are tightly controlled at 70 to 85 µmol/L [24,26].

With consumption of 5 to 9 servings of fruits and vegetables daily, steady-state plasma concentrations are 80 µmol/L or less, and peak values do not exceed 220 µmol/L, even after maximum oral administration of 3 g 6 times daily (18 g total) [38]. By contrast, intravenous vitamin C may produce plasma concentrations as high as 15000 µmol/L [27].

In human beings, the intestinal absorption is efficient and occurs along the entire length of the human intestine [3], mainly in the duodenum [11]. Intestinal absorption of vitamin C is by an active, sodium-dependent, energy-requiring, carrier-mediated transport mechanism [39] and as intake increases, the tissues become progressively more saturated. The physiologically efficient, renal-tubular reabsorption mechanism retains vitamin C in the tissues up to a whole-body content of ascorbate of about 20 mg/kg body weight [40]. However, under steady-state conditions, as intake rises from around 100 mg/day there is an increase in urinary output so that at 1000 mg/day almost all absorbed vitamin C is excreted [41,42].

A dynamic flow model for vitamin C has been postulated by Hickey et al. [43]. In their study, it is stated that the plasma ascorbate levels corresponding to varying intakes of ascorbate exhibit dual-phase pharmacokinetics. The first phase occurs when blood levels are below 70 μmol/L (0,123 mg/dl). In this stage, the kidney's vitamin C transporters reabsorb ascorbate [43-45]. While the ascorbate concentration remains relatively low, the transporters pump ascorbate back into the blood stream preventing its loss by renal clearance. The switch toward a second stage begins when the blood ascorbate concentration reaches 70 μmol/L, and the body excretes ascorbate more rapidly [46].

It is important to remark that differently to typical drugs, the half-life of vitamin C depends on its plasma levels. Accordingly, when plasma levels are above 70 μmol/L, ascorbate has a half-life of about 30 minutes [27]. However, in periods of deficient intake, when the renal transporters actively reabsorb the vitamin preventing acute scurvy, the plasma half-life of ascorbate is widely reported to be between 8 to 40 days [13,40]. Therefore, in healthy subjects, large doses taken several hours apart should be considered independent, as should be their bioavailability. From this pattern follows that splitting a single large dose into several smaller ones, taken a few hours apart, increases the effective bioavailability of the large dose.

Regarding absolute bioavailability, from 70 to 90 percent of usual dietary intakes of ascorbic acid (30 to 180 mg/day) are absorbed [13], although absorption decreases to about 50 percent and less with single doses above 1 g [24,40]. The type of food consumed has not been shown to have a significant effect on absorption of either intrinsic or supplemental vitamin C [13]. The relative bioavailability of pure synthetic ascorbic acid has not been shown to be significantly different from that of the vitamin naturally found in foods or in the form of a supplement [47,48].

Nevertheless, Cathcart's bowel tolerance method indicates that individual absorption and thus, bioavailability, can vary by a factor of at least two orders of magnitude, hence confirming that any variation depends upon the individual's health status [49]. Accordingly, bioavailability is not a static property of ascorbate, but it is subject to individual differences and varies with the timing of the dose. It follows that the appropriate intake will vary widely, both between individuals and also over time for the same person, depending on factors such as state of health and intake patterns, among others.

In addition, the oral bioavailability estimates reported in the literature may be somewhat biased because they are frequently based on the assumption that the rate of ascorbate absorption is linear and therefore the non-linear carrier-mediated absorption is often ignored. Likewise, multiple oral doses are expected to produce fluctuations in the absorption rate. Despite the uncertainty in the estimation of oral bioavailability, the analysis suggests that plasma ascorbate concentrations largely depend on limited absorption, probably as a result of a saturable transport mechanism.

Because ascorbate absorption is mediated by transport sites in the proximal small intestine, factors that reduce the rate at which the concentration of ascorbate builds up at these carrier sites (e.g., a delay in the rate of stomach emptying or a modified drug delivery system) would be expected to increase the absorbed fraction. Indeed, the bioavailability of ascorbate will be increased when given in divided doses or concurrently with food [50].

Ascorbate distribution volume has been reported ranging from 19.9 to 27 liters [51,52], which seems to be a reasonable value for a water-soluble vitamin.

Accordingly, evidence shows that some cell types actively accumulate ascorbate amounts above the actual plasma levels due to the fact that they have critical requirements for ascorbate and/or increased ascorbate transporters (Figure 2). As an example, urinary loss of ascorbate decreases ascorbate concentrations in plasma and in most tissues, but not the brain [53]. This might be related to the fact ascorbate plays a key role in neurotransmission in the brain, and that the transporters create a micro-environment in this tissue due to the cerebrospinal fluid (CSF). According to Hickey et al. [43], both white and red blood cells should be considered as specialized corporal reservoirs for ascorbate uptake from the blood supply, so that the mean and minimum blood levels become of cardinal interest to its availability [27].

Vitamin C is actively secreted in human gastric juice. Proton pump inhibitor therapy lowers the concentration of vitamin C in gastric juice and the proportion of the vitamin in its active antioxidant form i.e., ascorbic acid.

There is also some evidence that proton pump inhibitors may reduce the bioavailability of ingested vitamin C. The effect of proton pump inhibitors on vitamin C is more marked in *Helicobacter pylori*-infected subjects [54].

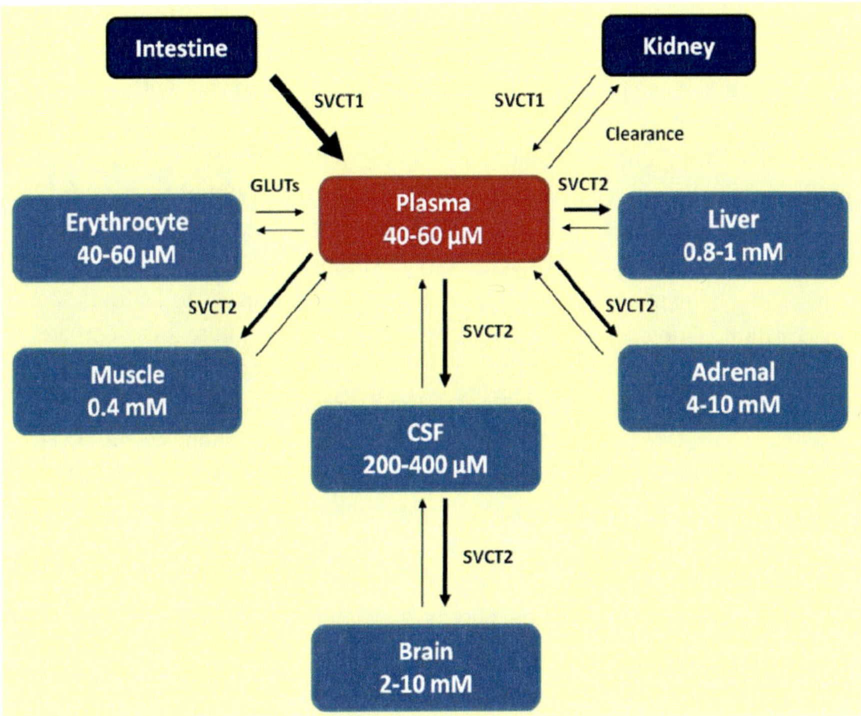

Figure 2. Relationships among intestinal absorption, plasma ascorbate and tissue accumulation. The kidney plays a two-sided role: it can eliminate ascorbate by clearance or it can pump it back into the blood, according to requirements determined by plasma concentration. SVTC1 / 2: sodium-dependent vitamin C transporters 1 and 2, GLUTs: facilitated glucose transporters of the GLUT family.

D. Transport and Metabolism

Vitamin C is one of the most important water soluble antioxidants in mammalian tissues. Its role as a free radical scavenger and its redox relationship with other antioxidants has been the focus of continuous interest. However, less attention has been paid to the metabolism of ascorbate, whose mechanisms are not yet fully understood, and sometimes the fact that humans are unable to synthesize the vitamin diverted the interest in this area.

Remarkably, some authors believe that the exploration of ascorbate metabolism and its regulation may contribute to the understanding of the evolutionary event leading to the loss of ascorbate synthesizing capability.

The ascorbate utilizing reactions are based on its property of being easily oxidized to dehydroascorbate. Ascorbate can be regenerated from its oxidized dehydroascorbate form (NADPH-dependent ascorbate recycling) in any mammalian cell of species [55]. Economically, it is more advantageous for the cell to reduce back the oxidized form of ascorbate than to synthesize it *de novo*. This recycling mechanism could therefore be interpreted as a phylogenetically gained adaptive benefit in superior mammalian species [27].

In species unable to synthesize ascorbate, the breakdown of the exogenous ascorbate can fuel the Cori cycle both in the liver and in the periphery. The uptake mechanism can be different in various cells, but some features seem to be constant. Considering the water soluble ionized nature of ascorbate and dehydroascorbate, simple diffusion through plasma membrane is often considered to play a minor role in tissue uptake. A facilitated mechanism involving a protein transporter has been postulated by Banhegyi et al. [55].

Intracellular ascorbate concentrations in the low millimolar range (much higher than that in plasma) seem to be necessary to support its role as an antioxidant [56] and as a cofactor for dioxygenase enzymes [57,58]. Whereas multiple intracellular recycling mechanisms help to maintain high intracellular ascorbate levels, sodium- and energy-dependent transport of the vitamin is necessary to achieve a concentration gradient from blood or the interstitium into cells.

I. Transport

The trans-plasma membrane gradient of ascorbate is generated by specific ascorbate transporters that were first cloned in 1999 [59]. Two isoforms of these transporters are known, and although similar in amino acid sequence and structure, they have different tissue distributions [59]. Both transporters mediate high-affinity, sodium- and energy-dependent ascorbate transport into cells and, as noted above, are essential to establish steep concentration gradients of the vitamin across the plasma membrane [59]. The nomenclature for both isoforms has evolved since the cloning of the protein in 1999 [59].

The sodium-dependent vitamin C transporter type 1 (SVCT1; product of the SLC23A1 gene in humans) is a voltage-dependent and rheogenic two Na^+-one L-ascorbate$^-$ cotransporter (symporter) with high affinity for L-ascorbic acid ($K_m \approx 70$ μmol/L) [5]. A broad range has been reported recently, 65–237 μmol/L [3].

SVCT1 resides largely in apical brushborder membranes of intestinal and renal tubular cells, where it helps to mediate absorption and reabsorption of the vitamin, respectively. Its absence in a knockout mouse has recently been shown to impair renal ascorbate reabsorption [60].

The human SVCT1 is a Na^+-dependent transporter that favors L-ascorbic acid over D-isoascorbic acid and that the oxidized form of vitamin C, dehydroascorbic acid, is excluded [44,61].

Na^+-L-ascorbic acid coupling stoichiometry has recently been determined [5] by measuring $^{22}Na^+$ and L-[^{14}C]ascorbic acid fluxes in individual oocytes under voltage clamp and relating the fluxes to net charge translocation. Two Na^+were transported per net positive charge, and the net positive charge influx was equivalent to the influx of L-ascorbic acid. Because L-ascorbic acid bears a charge of 1- at pH 7.5, these data demonstrated that the coupling ratio is two Na^+per one L-ascorbic acid under the conditions described. The Hill coefficient (n_H Na^+) for $Na^+ \approx 2$, thus indicating there is strong cooperativity between the two Na^+-binding sites involved in cotransport.

The SVCT2 (product of the SLC23A2 gene in humans), on the other hand, is found in cells of most other tissues [59]. This transporter is especially important in the brain.

Interestingly, targeted deletion of the widely distributed SVCT2 is lethal in mice [62], further underlining the importance of vitamin C.

In most non-neuronal cell types, the SVCT2 has a high affinity for ascorbate ($K_m \approx$ 8–62 μmol/L [3]). This affinity corresponds to plasma ascorbate concentrations of 30–60 μM. However, the apparent K_m for ascorbate transport in cultured neuroblastoma cells is somewhat higher, being by 100–110 μM [63,64], which correlates to higher CSF and interstitial ascorbate concentrations (200–400 μM) that supply the neurons with ascorbate. Even if this relationship holds for the neuronal SVCT2 *in vivo*, the neuronal ascorbate transporter will still be nearly saturated by extracellular ascorbate.

The latter suggests that ascorbate uptake and content in neurons will be limited by the number of SVCT2 expressed proteins, and affinity for ascorbate becomes relevant only when ascorbate deficiency is present [53]. Indeed, vitamin C is accumulated in some cells in part by the sodium-dependent transporter with saturable kinetics [27]. Ascorbic acid is concentrated in adrenal gland, pituitary, liver, spleen, and brain [65,66]. These organs have the greatest retention capacities. In brain, ascorbic acid accumulates mainly in cortex, nucleus accumbens, hypothalamus, hippocampus, and choroid plexus [67-69].

It has been proposed that in the presence of extracellular Na^+, the transporter was fully functional in the absence of either Ca^{2+} or Mg^{2+}, but there was no transport in the simultaneous absence of both cations. In the absence of extracellular Na^+, there was no transport irrespective of the absence or the presence of Ca^{2+} or Mg^{2+}. Thus, either Ca^{2+} or Mg^{2+} is essential for the function of SVCT2, which therefore can be defined as a bivalent cation-dependent transporter. On the other hand, the binding of Na^+ induces a transition in the transporter from a low to a high affinity conformation, which indicates that SVCT2 is activated by Na^+, but it is not a Na^+-dependent transporter [70].

It has been established a simultaneous transport model with binding sequence Na^+, L-ascorbic acid, Na^+ for the SVCT1 [5] (Figure 3). The same binding sequence was recently proposed for a second SVCT isoform, human SVCT2 [70]. However, in the latter study, the evidence cited does not seem to support that conclusion, rather, for a simultaneous transport mechanism, and V_{max} data provided elsewhere in that study may instead support the binding sequence Na^+, Na^+, L-ascorbic acid for SVCT2 [5].

The two Na^+-dependent transporters can be subjected to fine-tuned regulation by their own substrate. An elevated level of ascorbate in the intestinal lumen leads to down-regulation of SVCT1 mRNA in enterocytes [71]. A similar self-regulatory role for ascorbate was demonstrated for SVCT2 in platelets [72]. Recently, it was shown that skeletal muscle cells modulated the expression of the SVCT2 carrier according to their redox balance in order to preserve redox homeostasis. Both mRNA and protein levels of SVCT2 were up-regulated in hydrogen peroxide-treated myotubes, while antioxidant supplementation with lipoic acid lowered the expression of SVCT2 [73]. It seems likely that the redox state of the cell can influence the expression of SVCT2 and thus, the resulting response regulates the transport and intracellular level of ascorbate.

In addition to ascorbate uptake through the SVCT proteins, DHA can enter and leave cells by facilitated diffusion on the ubiquitous glucose transporters of the GLUT family (GLUTs). Surprisingly, the same as the SVCT1 excludes DHA, ascorbate is not transported by the GLUTs [74]. The characteristics of DHA uptake by luminal membranes of the human jejunum clearly differ from those of ascorbate uptake [75]. DHA is taken up by low-affinity (K_m 1–4 mmol/L; [74,76,77]) sodium-independent facilitated diffusion. The transport protein responsible for the intestinal absorption of DHA has not yet been identified [3].

DHA forms a bicyclic hemiketal in solution [78,79] (Figure 4), which is likely the species transported by the GLUTs [80]. DHA is transported by glucose transporters, particularly GLUT1, GLUT3 and GLUT4 [81], and is therefore not energetically driven. The evidence regarding GLUT2 is still controversial, and there are no data regarding the capacity of GLUT8, GLUT10, and GLUT12–GLUT14 to transport dehydroascorbic acid. GLUT5 is a fructose transporter unable to transport dehydroascorbic acid, which is probably also the situation with GLUT7, GLUT9, and GLUT11, although these last transporters have been less studied from a functional perspective [70].

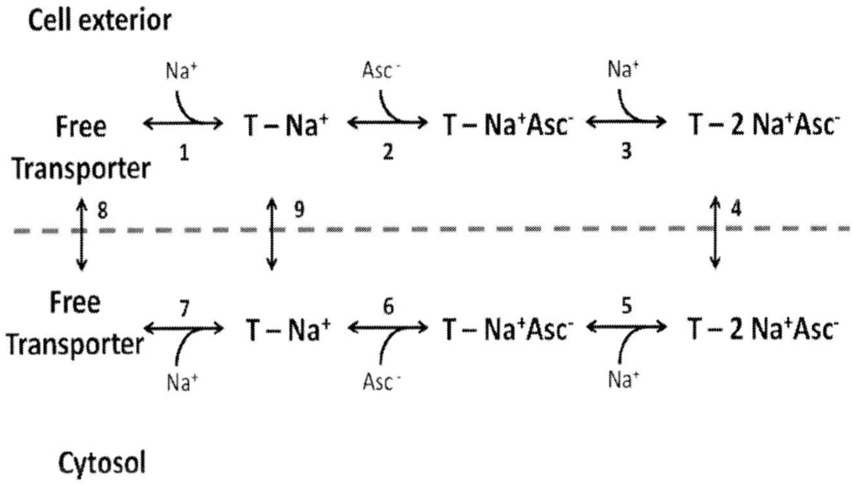

Figure 3. The binding sequence for the SVCT1, as an 8 step transport. 1, 2, 3: ordered loading of a free transporter with sodium, then ascorbate and finally sodium. 4: trans-membrane transport. 5, 6, 7: ordered liberation of sodium, then ascorbate to end with sodium. 8: the transporter becomes functional again. 9: it has also been demonstrated a minor "internal leakage", with the sole transport of one sodium [5].

Intracellular DHA is readily converted to ascorbate and this highly favorable reductive step drives DHA uptake by the cell. Nonetheless, DHA uptake and reduction could well preserve intracellular ascorbate over short time periods in areas of high oxidative stress, where significant amounts of extracellular ascorbate are oxidized [82].

Notably, the rapid reduction of dehydroascorbate on the internal side of plasma membrane by various reducing systems prevents the efflux of this compound and allows the effective accumulation of ascorbate against a concentration gradient as it has been observed in several cell types [27].

There are also mechanisms allowing the efflux of ascorbate from cells [75], e.g. from enterocytes during intestinal absorption and from liver cells, which produces ascorbate in many mammals – excluding humans –, but the molecular identity of the proteins involved in this process is not yet firmly established.

Whereas ascorbate can efflux from various cell types [83,84], including neurons [85], because of its hydrophilic nature and negative charge at physiologic pH, it does over several hours in the absence of an efflux mechanism [86].

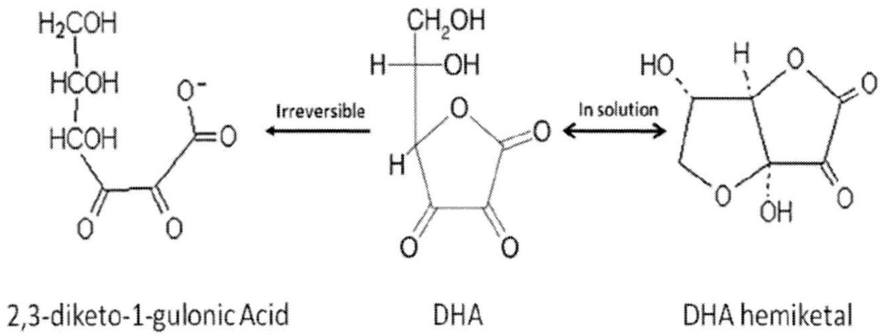

Figure 4. Some metabolic pathways concerning DHA: DHA hemiketal in solution as transported by the GLUTs and irreversible conversion to 2,3-diketo-1-gulonic acid to follow elimination.

II. Metabolism

This part of the chapter will refer to the recycling of vitamin C inside the cell and its degradation. For a general view of the reactions of ascorbate in relation to its functions refer to the Biological Functions section.

II.1. Recycling of Vitamin C

As described in the introduction, ascorbate plays a major role as a water-soluble antioxidant and as a cofactor of several enzymes, which lead to its one electron oxidation to SDA. Disproportionation of SDA (2 SDA → ascorbate + DHA), in turn, results in the formation of DHA (Fig 5.). If SDA accumulates significantly in areas not accessible to the enzymes, or if its concentration exceeds their capacity, two molecules of SDA react or dismutate to form one molecule each of ascorbate and dehydroascorbic acid (DHA) [87].

Both SDA and DHA are reduced back to ascorbate by several enzymatic systems that are briefly reviewed below and schematized in Figure 5.

II.2. Reduction of Semidehydroascorbate

The reduction of SDA in the cytosol has been assigned to enzymes using NADH (NADH-cytochrome b5 reductase) or NADPH (thioredoxin reductase). SDA can also be reduced in the lumen of neuroendocrine secretory vesicles or in the external medium by transmembrane electron transfer systems [37].

NADH-Cytochrome B5 Reductase

Early studies showed that oxidation of NADH by liver microsomes was stimulated in the presence of SDA, and microsomal NADH-cytochrome b5 reductase was proposed to participate in the electron transfer system, since the purified enzyme itself was able to reduce SDA in the presence of NADH [88].

Thioredoxin Reductase

Purified rat liver thioredoxin reductase, a selenoprotein, was shown to catalyze the NADPH-dependent reduction of SDA with a Km value (in the presence of thioredoxin, which acts as an activator) of $\approx$ 3 µmol/L for this radical [89].

Cytochrome B561-Mediated Reduction of Intravesicular SDA

Ascorbate is a cofactor of dopamine β-hydroxylase and of peptidylglycine α-amidating monooxygenase. Both enzymes are confined to a small area in neuroendocrine secretory vesicles (catecholamine-storing vesicles for the first enzyme and peptide-storing vesicles for the second) and catalyze reactions generating SDA [90]. As ascorbate and SDA do not cross the membrane of the storage vesicles, the reduction of SDA to ascorbate occurs inside the vesicles and involves the transmembrane transfer of electrons by cytochrome b561, the second most abundant protein in the chromaffin granule membrane [91]. Electrons are furnished to cytochrome b561 by cytosolic ascorbate, which is maintained under its reduced form by the mitochondrial outer membrane SDA reductase [92]. The intravesicular reduction of SDA to ascorbate is thermodynamically driven by the pH gradient (SDA reduction involves the binding of a proton and is therefore favoured at acidic pH) and the membrane potential (positive inside) created across the chromaffin vesicle membrane by an inwardly directed proton translocating ATPase [93].

II.3. Reduction of Extracellular SDA Involving Transfer of Electrons Across the Plasma Membrane

Erythrocytes are able to transfer electrons from intracellular donors to extracellular SDA. In a system where SDA was generated extracellularly from ascorbate by ascorbate oxidase, it was shown that erythrocytes decreased both the ascorbate oxidation rate and the steady-state extracellular SDA concentration [94]. It does not involve cytochrome b561, which is absent from the erythrocyte plasma membrane [95].

II.4. Reduction of Dehydroascorbate

This process is probably less important quantitatively than the reduction of SDA, which is the most important oxidation product of ascorbate. Intracellular DHA may, however, derive from SDA through disproportionation or through import from extracellular sources. This process may be of particular importance for the administration of DHA in pathophysiological conditions.

Spontaneous Reaction with Gluthathione (GSH)

DHA can be non-enzymatically reduced to ascorbate by GSH [96]. This reaction, which presumably proceeds through a glutathione-ascorbate thiohemiketal adduct, is thermodynamically favourable, but is relatively slow at physiological concentrations of GSH.

However, as detailed below, several enzymes facilitate this reaction with GSH. Furthermore, NADPH-dependent reductases appear also to be involved in DHA reduction.

Glutaredoxin

Highly purified preparations of glutaredoxin display DHA reductase activity [97]. Glutaredoxin is a thiol-disulfide oxidoreductase, which possesses active-site cysteine residues.

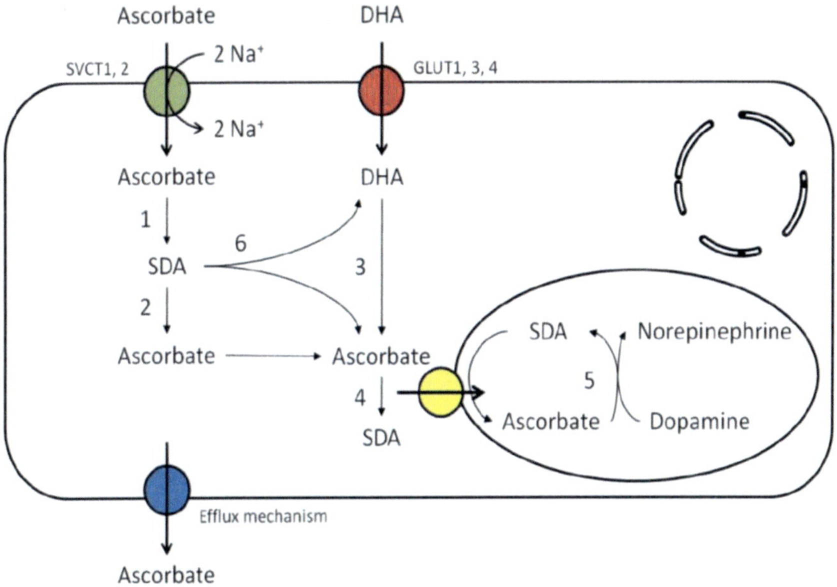

Figure 5. Brief schematic including transport and metabolism of vitamin C. Ascorbate and DHA are transported by the SVCTs and GLUTs respectively. 1: ascorbate reduces biomolecules such as vitamin E and reactive oxygen species. 2: SDA is reduced back to ascorbate by NAD(P)H-dependent enzymes. 3: DHA is reduced back to ascorbate by gluthathione or NAD(P)H-dependent enzymes. It is also self-reduced by gluthathione. 4: electrons are furnished into the mitochondria. 5: the furnished electrons are then utilized in catecholamine synthesis. 6: accumulation of SDA leads to disproportionation and conversion of equimolar ascorbate and DHA.

II.5. Degradation of Vitamin C in Mammals

In Vivo Studies

In human subjects injected with ascorbate labelled on C1, an average of 44% of the total radioactivity excreted in urine was recovered as oxalate; other urinary metabolites were 2,3-diketo-L-gulonic acid (2,3-DKG) (≈20%) and DHA (< 2%), and ≈20% of the total urinary radioactivity was present as ascorbate [98]. Little if any radioactivity was recovered as CO2.

Spontaneous Breakdown of Dehydroascorbate

Ascorbate is oxidized to DHA in a variety of enzymatic and nonenzymatic reactions. DHA can be reduced back to ascorbate, but can also be hydrolyzed to 2,3-diketo-L-gulonate (2,3-DKG) (Figure 4). The latter reaction is irreversible and 2,3-DKG, unlike DHA, is therefore devoid of antiscorbutic activity. DHA is unstable and nonenzymatic hydrolysis occurs rather rapidly at neutral pH, the half-time of decay being about 5–15 min at 37 °C [99]. Incubation of DHA or 2,3-DKG in the presence of phosphate buffer (pH 7) for several hours at 37 °C leads to the formation of L-erythrulose and oxalate [100], indicating cleavage between the second and the third carbon [37]. The latter is the two-electron-oxidized form of ascorbate, which is very unstable, having a half-life in blood and physiologic buffers of 2–6 min [101,102].

E. Biological Functions

Despite most investigations on the health-protective effects of vitamins C have been focused merely on its antioxidant power, this compound represents one of the most fascinating natural resources that have the potential to influence a broad range of mechanisms underlying human health and disease. Hence, the biological properties of ascorbic acid have overwhelmed its antioxidant effects.

Vitamin C is an electron donor and therefore a reducing agent. In all of its known functions, ascorbate serves as a one-electron donor, generating semidehydroascorbate. When ascorbate acts as an antioxidant or enzyme cofactor, it becomes oxidized to dehydroascorbic acid [101]. The latter can be used by cells to regenerate ascorbate, and directly or indirectly, it can change the redox state of many other molecules [103].

Vitamin C Antioxidant Effect

Vitamin C counteracts and prevents the oxidation of lipids, proteins and DNA, subsequently protecting their structure and biological function. The oxidation of these biomolecules generates measurable reaction products, such as 8-hydroxy-2-deoxyguanosine from DNA [104], F2-isoprostanes from lipids [105], and carbonyl derivatives from proteins [106]. Moreover, this can give a useful method to assess the antioxidant effect of vitamin C or other antioxidants. In addition, the generation of ascorbyl radical has been used to monitor the extent of oxidative stress using electron paramagnetic resonance spectroscopy in patients with sepsis [107].

Ascorbate in aqueous compartments can recycle α-tocopherol in membranes by reducing the α-tocopheroxyl radical back to α-tocopherol

(Figure 6). Indeed, ascorbate has been shown to spare/recycle α-tocopherol in lipid bilayers [108] and in erythrocytes [109], therefore, enhancing vitamin E antioxidant properties. It has been shown that antioxidative action of α - tocopherol results in its oxidation to the toxic radical α-tocopheroxyl. The regeneration of α-tocopherol, which restores its antioxidative properties, is promoted by vitamin C [110]. This is of particular importance to interpret the results of several studies aiming cardiovascular protection utilizing vitamin E alone.

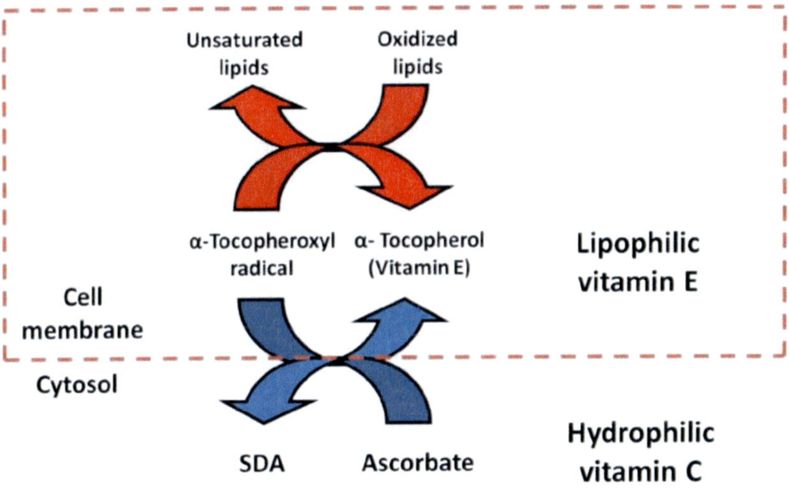

Figure 6. Vitamin C recycles vitamin E in the water-lipid interface.

Given the lipid-rich environment of the brain, the sparing or recycling of α-tocopherol may be a very important role for ascorbate. Accordingly, when ascorbate is added to cultured cells, brain slices, and brain microsomes it prevents lipid peroxidation induced by various oxidizing agents [111], especially in combination with α-tocopherol [112].

Ascorbate directly scavenges oxygen- or nitrogen-based radical species generated during normal cellular metabolism [53]. The major radical byproduct of mitochondrial oxygen metabolism is superoxide [113]. Although ascorbate concentrations of 100 μM and higher are required to appreciably scavenge superoxide [56], ascorbate concentrations in nucleated cells are typically in the low millimolar range [113]. At the millimolar concentrations present in neurons *in vivo*, ascorbate will effectively scavenge superoxide [56], a major diffusible byproduct of rapid neuronal mitochondrial metabolism, oxidative stress and ischemia-reperfusion [114]. *In vivo* studies outline a more convincing role for an antioxidant effect of ascorbate in brain, especially those dealing with ischemia–reperfusion [53].

For a brief review of oxide-reductive pathways regarding vitamin C, refer to Figure 7.

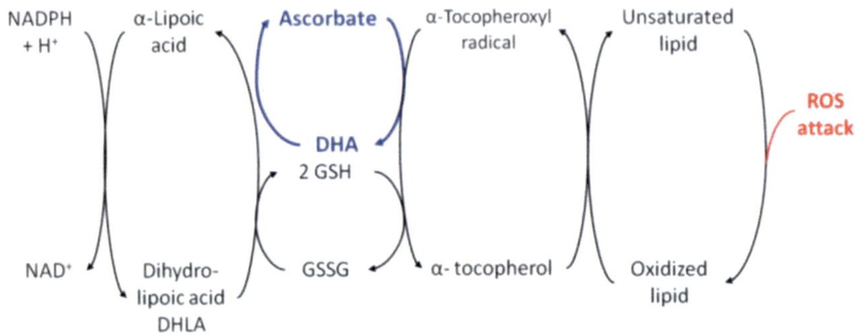

Figure 7. Ascorbate, as a cornerstone in oxide-reductive systems in the cell.

Enzymatic Functions

Vitamin C acts as an electron donor for numerous human enzymes: three participate in collagen hydroxylation [115] and two in carnitine biosynthesis [116]; of the three enzymes which participate in collagen hydroxylation, one is necessary for biosynthesis of the catecholamine norepinephrine [117], another is necessary for amidation of peptide hormones [118,119], and the last is involved in tyrosine metabolism [120]. Ascorbate interacts with enzymes having either monooxygenase or dioxygenase activity. The monooxygenases, dopamine β-monooxygenase and peptidyl-glycine α-monooxygenase, incorporate a single oxygen atom into a substrate, either a dopamine or a glycine-terminating peptide. The dioxygenases incorporate two oxygen atoms in two different ways: the enzyme 4-hydroxyphenylpyruvate dioxygenase incorporates two oxygen atoms into one product; the other dioxygenase incorporates one oxygen atom into succinate and one into the enzyme-specific substrate [7].

Of course, vitamin C best-known function is to facilitate the hydroxylation of proline and lysine residues in collagen, allowing proper intracellular folding of procollagen for export and deposition as mature collagen [53]. Given the clinical manifestations of scurvy (hemorrhage, loss of teeth, tendon rupture), stabilization of collagen by ascorbate certainly seems to be critical to forming the connective tissue framework of the entire body; including skin, bones, cartilage, tendons, ligaments, and blood vessels [113].

Functions of Vitamin C in the Brain

The functions of ascorbate in the central nervous system (CNS) and brain are numerous [53]. Although all actions of ascorbate involve the donation of a single electron, they can be divided into those considered antioxidant and non-antioxidant in nature. Many of the latter functions involve monovalent reduction of Fe^{3+} or Cu^{2+} at the active sites of dioxygenase enzymes in hydroxylation reactions.

Together with the antioxidant functions, ascorbate performs non-antioxidant functions in brain and neural-derived tissues, centered on neurotransmitters. For example, it is well established that ascorbate is essential for catecholamine biosynthesis in neural tissues, serving as a cofactor for dopamine β-hydroxylase in the conversion of dopamine to norepinephrine [117,121]. Moreover, several groups have documented a novel mechanism involving ascorbate and SDA to enable the transfer of electrons across the chromaffin granule membrane [122,123].

Ascorbate inside the granule is oxidized to SDA, either in hydroxylation reactions or in simply scavenging radicals that might otherwise react with redox-sensitive catechols in the granule. This SDA is then reduced back to ascorbate by interaction with the reduced form of a cytochrome b561 in the granule membrane, which is maintained in the reduced form by accepting an electron from cytoplasmic ascorbate. Ascorbate in chromaffin granules is then secreted concomitantly with catecholamines from cultured chromaffin cells [124] and in vivo by human adrenal glands, the latter in response to adrenocorticotrophin stimulation [125].

Ascorbate has been proposed to function as a neuromodulator of both dopamine- and glutamate-mediated neurotransmission [85]. More recent studies relating ascorbate modulation of glutamate dynamics with changes in rat behavior show that such modulation is complex, because it depends on the studied site in the brain, level of behavioral activity, and level of extracellular ascorbate [126-128]. The mechanism(s) by which ascorbate affects neuronal transmission has not been established, but they could be related in part to redox changes in the N-methyl-D-aspartate (NMDA) receptor. For example, ascorbate has been shown to protect neurons from excitotoxicity induced by activation of the NMDA receptor and it prevented glutamate-induced cell damage and death in cultured cerebellar granule cells [129,130]. This could be due to redox modulation of the receptor itself by ascorbate [131] or to direct scavenging of ROS generated by receptor activation. A more severe stress of ischemia releases large amounts of ascorbate from brain cells [132], what is associated with glutamate uptake by neurons and glia [133]. Removal of extracellular glutamate by such a process would also decrease excitotoxicity caused by activation of cell surface and synaptic glutamate receptors [134].

There is also evidence that ascorbate is involved in the regulation of both acetylcholine and catecholamine release from synaptic vesicles [135]. Furthermore, ascorbate has been shown to be an effective acetylcholinesterase inhibitor [136].

In addition to the noted effects of ascorbate on neurotransmitters, ascorbate has been shown to be involved in neuropeptide amidation [118,119] and release in the brain [137].

Ascorbate-dependent collagen synthesis has also been linked to formation of the myelin sheath that surrounds many neuronal processes: ascorbate added to a mixed culture of rat Schwann cells and dorsal root ganglion neurons promoted myelin formation and differentiation by Schwann cells during formation of the basal lamina of the myelin sheath [138]. The latter process was considered linked to the ability of the Schwann cells to generate collagen.

Other Functions

Vitamin C behaves as a blood pressure modulator on the vascular wall, exerting up-regulation on endothelial NO synthase (eNOS) and downregulation of NADPH oxidase [139]. Recently, it was demonstrated that vitamin C inhibits the effects of endothelin-1 (ET-1) of impairing endothelium-dependent and endothelium-independent vasodilation and the stimulation of interleukin-6 (IL-6) release in humans *in vivo* [103]. This suggested that the mechanism by which ET-1 impairs vascular function and stimulates release of IL-6 involves increased oxidative stress [140]. Another cardiovascular function of ascorbate is that it protects low-density lipoproteins ex vivo against oxidation and may function similarly in the blood [141].

Ascorbate has also been shown to assist other prolyl and lysyl hydroxylases in the hydroxylation of hypoxia-inducible factor 1α (HIF-1α). HIF-1α is a transcription factor responsible for the cellular response to low-oxygen conditions through activation of genes controlling diverse cellular pathways, including glycolysis, iron transport, angiogenesis, and cell survival [142]. Hydroxylation of HIF-1α targets it for destruction in the proteasome, thereby down-regulating the pathways dependent on transcriptional regulation by hypoxia.

Concentrations of vitamin C appear to be high in gastric juice. Schorah et al. [143] found that the concentrations of vitamin C in gastric juice were severalfold higher (median, 249 mmol/l; range, 43–909 mmol/l) than those found in the plasma of the same normal subjects (median, 39 mmol/l; range, 14–101 mmol/l). Gastric juice vitamin C may prevent the formation of N-nitroso compounds, which are potentially mutagenic [144]. High intakes of vitamin C correlate with reduced gastric cancer risk [145], but a cause-and-effect relationship has not been established.

A common feature of vitamin C deficiency is anemia. Vitamin C high levels in the stomach may be useful to promote absorption of soluble non-haem iron possibly by chelation or simply by maintaining the iron in the reduced (ferrous, Fe^{2+}) form [146]. This effect can be achieved with the amounts of vitamin C obtained in foods. However, the amount of dietary vitamin C required to increase iron absorption ranges from 25 mg upwards and depends largely on the amount of inhibitors, such as phytates and polyphenols, present in the meal [147]. The antioxidant properties of vitamin C may also play a role in anemia. Ascorbate stabilizes folate in food and in plasma; increased excretion of oxidized folate derivatives in humans with scurvy has been reported [148].

Chapter III

Consequences of Vitamin C Deficiency

From the 15th century, scurvy was dreaded by seamen and explorers forced to subsist for months on diets of dried beef and biscuits. Scurvy was described by the Crusaders during the sieges of numerous European cities, and was also a result of the famine in 19th century Ireland.

Three important manifestations of scurvy—gingival changes, pain in the extremities, and haemorrhagic manifestations—precede oedema, ulcerations, and ultimately death. Skeletal and vascular lesions related to scurvy probably arise from a failure of osteoid formation. In infantile scurvy the changes are mainly at the sites of most active bone growth; characteristic signs are a pseudoparalysis of the limbs caused by extreme pain on movement and caused by haemorrhages under the periosteum, as well as swelling and haemorrhages of the gums surrounding erupting teeth [149]. In adults, one of the early principle adverse effects of the collagen-related pathology may be impaired wound healing [150].

Vitamin C deficiency can be detected from early signs of clinical deficiency, such as the follicular hyperkeratosis, petechial haemorrhages, swollen or bleeding gums, and joint pain, or from the very low concentrations of ascorbate in plasma, blood, or leukocytes.

The Sheffield studies [150,151] and the later studies in Iowa [152,153] were the first major attempts to quantify vitamin C requirements. The studies indicated that the amount of vitamin C required to prevent or cure early signs of deficiency ranges between 6.5 and 10 mg/day. This range represents the lowest physiological requirement. The Iowa studies [152,153] and Kallner et al. [40] established that at tissue saturation, whole-body vitamin C content is approximately 20 mg/kg, or 1500 mg, and that during depletion vitamin C is lost at a rate of 3% of whole-body content per day. Clinical signs of scurvy appear in men at intakes lower than 10 mg/day [151] or when the whole-body content falls below 300 mg [152]. Such intakes are associated with plasma ascorbate concentrations below 11 μmol/L or leukocyte levels less than 2 nmol/10^8 cells. However, plasma concentrations fall to about 11 μmol/L even when dietary vitamin C is between 10 and 20 mg/day. At intakes greater than 25–35 mg/day, plasma concentrations start to rise steeply, indicating a greater availability of vitamin C for metabolic needs [7].

In general, plasma ascorbate closely reflects the dietary intake and ranges between 20 and 80 μmol/L. During infection or physical trauma, the number of circulating leukocytes increases and these take up vitamin C from the plasma [154]. Therefore, both plasma and leukocyte levels may not be very precise indicators of body content or status at such times. However, leukocyte ascorbate remains a better indicator of vitamin C status than plasma ascorbate most of the time [7].

Populations at Risk of Vitamin C Deficiency

The populations at risk of vitamin C deficiency are those for whom the fruit and vegetable supply is minimal. Epidemics of scurvy are associated with famine and war, when people are forced to become refugees and food supply is small and irregular. Persons in whom the total body vitamin C content is saturated (i.e. 20 mg/kg body weight) can subsist without vitamin C for approximately 2 months before the appearance of clinical signs, and as little as 6.5–10 mg/day of vitamin C will prevent the appearance of scurvy. In general, vitamin C status will reflect the regularity of fruit and vegetable consumption; however, socioeconomic conditions are also factors as intake is determined not just by availability of food, but by cultural preferences and cost [7].

Chapter IV

Pathophysiology, Prevention and Treatment of Disease

The clinical use of antioxidants has gained considerable interest during the last decades. Indeed, vitamin C oral supplements are among the most popular sold, and gram doses are promoted for preventing and treating the common cold, managing stress, and enhancing well-being [155].

It was suggested from epidemiological studies that diets high in fruits and vegetables might help decrease the risk of cardiovascular disease. Therefore, vitamin supplements have been applied through protocols aimed to prevent diseases such as hypertension, atherosclerosis, preeclampsia or, among others, diseases thought to be mediated by oxidative stress. Despite the biological properties of these vitamins could account for an effective protection, as shown by several clinical and experimental studies, their efficacy remains controversial in the light of some recent clinical trials and meta-analyses [103].

As an example, low levels of vitamin C, have been associated not only with obesity [156] but also with a variety of conditions including hypertension, gallbladder disease, stroke, some cancers and atherosclerosis [157].

I. Hypertension

The elevation of blood pressure has been associated with ROS abundance and frequently also with an impairment of endogenous antioxidant mechanisms [158]. Thus, there is accumulating evidence that increased vascular oxidative stress could be involved in the pathogenesis of essential hypertension [159,160]. Most studies have demonstrated an inverse relationship between plasma ascorbate levels and blood pressure in both normotensive and hypertensive populations [161,162]. In addition, clinical studies have demonstrated that essential hypertensive patients produce excessive amount of ROS [163,164], as shown by their abnormal levels of antioxidant status [165]. Indeed, increased ROS production in vascular tissues, particularly superoxide anions, has been implicated as playing an important role in vascular events such as hypertension, vascular remodeling after angioplasty, atherosclerosis, myocardial infarction, and ischemic stroke [166].

ROS have multiple pathophysiological actions in the artery wall, including an impairment of endothelium-dependent vasodilation [167]. Superoxide is a major determinant of NO bioavailability and thus can modify endothelial function; it rapidly inactivates endothelium-derived NO, the most important endogenous vasodilator [168-170]. Thus, therapeutic strategies should aim to restore the bioavailability of NO, either scavenging ROS or through downregulation of their generation and/or upregulation of eNOS activity and antioxidant enzymes.

The major source of superoxide in the vascular wall is the enzyme NADPH oxidase, consisting of several membrane-bound subunits (gp91, Nox, and p22phox) and cytosolic subunits (p47phox, p67phox, p40phox, and Rac2) [171-173], an enzyme complex of vascular smooth muscle cells [174]. There appear to be at least three isoforms of NADPH oxidase expressed in the vascular wall. Thus, although endothelial cells and adventitial fibroblasts express a gp91phox-containing NADPH oxidase similar to that originally identified in phagocytes, vascular smooth muscle cells may rely on novel homologues of gp91phox, namely Nox1 and Nox4, to produce superoxide [160]. Upon assembly of the subunits in the membrane, this enzyme generates a burst of superoxide [171]. The most studied stimulus of the vascular NADPH oxidase is angiotensin II, although other pressor agents such as endothelin 1 and urotensin II are also involved, thereby resulting in increased ROS.

It was hypothesized that the pathological state of high blood pressure is associated with loss of balance between status of oxidative stress and level of antioxidants. Diminished antioxidant defense capacity has been well demonstrated in spontaneously hypertensive rats, associated with insufficient expression of all the three antioxidant enzymes [175].

An epidemiological study of the relationship of serum vitamin C concentration to the subsequent incidence of stroke, reported a negative association partly explained by lowering blood pressure [176,177].

Accordingly, numerous attempts to reinforce the antioxidant defense system have been made. Dietary intervention trials of the impact of high consumption of fruit and vegetables on antioxidant levels and blood pressure have demonstrated positive effects [178-180].

Treatment with antioxidants improves the vascular function and reduces the blood pressure in animal models [181,182] and in human hypertension [183,184]. Pharmacological doses of vitamin C produce vasodilation in the brachial and coronary arteries [41,185]. In healthy subjects, vitamin C administration restored endothelium-dependent vasodilation that was impaired by acute hyperglycemia [186], free fatty-acids [187], endotoxemia [188] and ischemia-reperfusion [189]. Also, in a recent study [190], N-acetylcysteine (NAC) showed no statistically significant effect on either endothelium-dependent or endothelium-independent vasodilation in essential hypertensive subjects, whereas vitamin C did.

Thus, vitamin C may have favorable effects on vascular dilation, possibly through its antioxidant effects on NO [191,56], but these findings are not consistent [192]. Moreover, in most studies, the vitamin C-induced effects on vasodilation occurred when vitamin C was administered intra-arterially [190].

In addition, both vitamin C and E not solely behave as ROS-scavengers, but also they are able to induce downregulation of NADPH oxidase and upregulation of endothelial eNOS [193]. The molecular mechanisms underlying the in vivo antioxidant effects of vitamin C related with blood pressure modulation are not fully understood. Nevertheless, it was shown that these effects are mediated in part by the ability of vitamin C to protect BH_4 from oxidation and thereby increase enzymatic activity of eNOS. It should be noted that BH_4 is a cofactor necessary for NO generation via eNOS, otherwise becoming uncoupled, a form now recognized as an important source of superoxide rather than NO [194,195], a condition likely to occur under a prooxidant state. Furthermore, ascorbic acid may reduce the α-tocopheroxyl radical and may be required for beneficial vascular effects of α-tocopherol [196]. In fact, the effect of α-tocopherol seems to be dependent on tissue saturation with vitamin C, and both vitamins may act synergistically to provide optimal conditions for endothelial NO formation [197].

Despite these biological effects of vitamin C and E, clinical long-term trials have failed to document consistently their beneficial effect in patients at high cardiovascular risk. In a recent study, a decreasing trend was observed with vitamin C levels and risk of hypertension in women but not in men [198]. Vitamin C supplementation is associated with reduced blood pressure in hypertensive patients, with systolic blood pressure falling by 3.6–17.8 mmHg for each 50 μmol/L increase in plasma ascorbate [161,192,199]. Nevertheless, there are several small and short-term clinical trials in which the effect of vitamin C supplements on blood pressure have yielded inconsistent findings [192,200-202]. The lack of antihypertensive efficacy observed in studies using supplementation with vitamin C alone could be due to the pharmacokinetics of vitamin C and/or the decreased bioavailability of NO under conditions of oxidative stress [203].

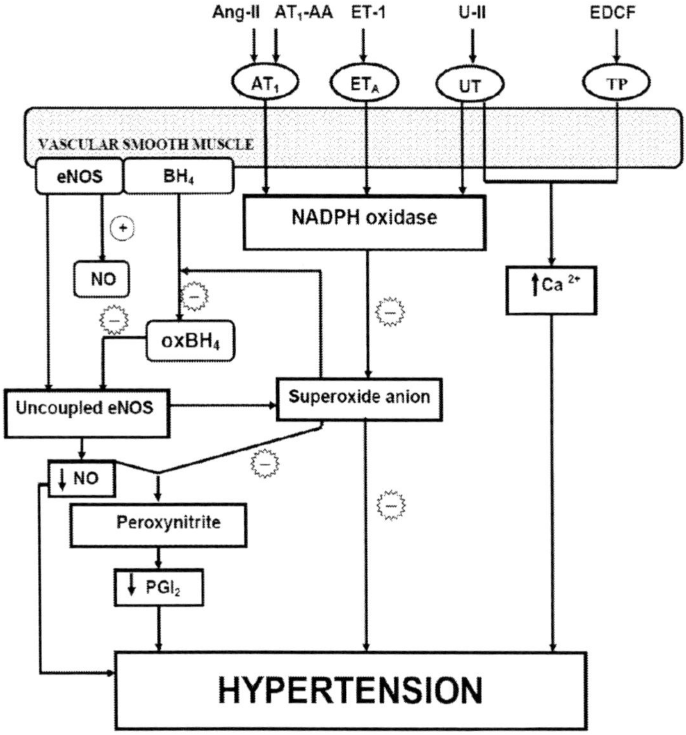

Figure 8. Involvement of vitamin C, as well as other antioxidants, in counteracting the elevation of blood pressure induced by oxidative stress. BH_4, tetrahydrobiopterin; $oxBH_4$, oxidized tetrahydrobiopterin; eNOS, endothelial nitric oxide synthase; NO, nitric oxide; Ang-II, angiotensin II; AT_1, angiotensin II type 1 receptors; AT_1-AA, autoantibodies to angiotensin II type 1 receptors; U-II, human urotensin II; UT, human urotensin II receptors; ET-1, endothelin-1; ET_A, type A endothelin-1 receptors; PGI_2, prostacyclin; EDCF, endothelium derived contracting factor; TP, thromboxane-prostaglandin receptors. The effects of vitamin C in these pathways are indicated as down-regulation (⊖) and up-regulation (⊕). From: Rodrigo R, 2009b [203], with permission.

The uncertain clinical beneficial effect of vitamin C and E in vivo as antihypertensive agents could be due to the lack of consideration of basic aspects such as their pharmacokinetic properties. Thus, it was experimentally determined that the antihypertensive effect of vitamin C is expected to occur at a concentration by 10 mmol/L [56], a plasma level unreachable in humans through oral administration, but that would be required to compete efficiently with the reaction of NO with superoxide, due to their high reaction rate constant, which is even higher than the reaction between superoxide dismutase (SOD) and NO [204].

The lack of a therapeutic antihypertensive plasma vitamin C concentration via oral administration may be due to its renal threshold in relation to the plasma concentration achievable by oral supplementation. The renal ascorbic acid threshold occurs at vitamin C doses between 60 and 100 mg daily. Plasma is completely saturated at doses of 400 mg daily and higher, producing a steady-state plasma concentration about 80 μmol/L [29]. Thus, the antihypertensive effect may only be active in plasma following vitamin C infusion at high doses. Recent pharmacokinetics modeling indicates that with oral administration, even at very large and frequent doses of vitamin C will increase plasma concentrations only modestly, from 70 μmol/L to a maximum of 220 μmol/L [38], whereas intravenous administration raises plasma concentrations as high as 15 mmol/L [27]. In addition, the fact that most of the clinical studies have been carried out without a detailed knowledge of the cellular functions of vitamins C and E, made an evaluation of epidemiological data more difficult. Hence, the available data are not conclusive and the relationship between blood pressure and antioxidant activity in humans has yet to be defined [103].

II. Atherosclerosis

Oxidative stress has been shown to play a central role in the development of atherosclerosis (Figure 9). The antioxidant functions of ascorbate may explain the observations of Willis over 50 years ago that both acute and chronic scurvy in guinea pigs produced intimal lesions indistinguishable from those of human atherosclerosis [205], and that such lesions were reversed by ascorbate supplements [206]. Indeed, atherosclerosis has been termed a disease of "latent" scurvy [207]. In this regard, it is intriguing to note that humans and guinea pigs (both unable to synthesize ascorbate) are the only mammals known to develop spontaneous atherosclerosis without dietary cholesterol feeding [207].

The oxidative stress-related detrimental events that could either trigger or exacerbate the atherosclerotic process include modification of proteins and DNA, alteration in gene expression, promotion of inflammation, and deterioration in endothelial function in the vessel wall [208-210]. The alteration in endothelial permeability due to endothelial injury causes transmigration of LDL particles into the intima, where these are modified by oxidative stress to oxidized LDL (oxLDL), potent chemoattractant for monocytes and T lymphocytes, and promotes the differentiation of monocytes to tissue macrophages. Consequently, the latter release various cytokines and initiate an inflammatory response in the initial stages of atherosclerosis [211].

oxLDL is an important mediator to cause plaque instability mainly by activating matrix metalloproteinases (MMP) [Xu et al., 1999], inducing the expression of macrophage scavenger receptor and thus promoting the foam cell formation [Stocker & Keaney, 2004]. Overproduction of ROS is associated with increased NADPH oxidase activity or eNOS uncoupling. The excessive ROS burden is thought to promote atherogenesis by exerting its effect at several steps, such as endothelial function, enhanced surface adhesion molecule expression, and LDL oxidation as well as MMP production and plaque rupture [211].

It is thought that the loss of endothelial function, a result of loss of eNOS activity and degradation of available NO, is followed by expression of adhesion molecules such as ICAM-1 and VCAM-1. The expression of endothelial cell surface receptors facilitates inflammatory cell recruitment and lipid deposition in the intimal layer. The subsequent ingestion of excess oxLDL particles by macrophages and monocytes results in inflammatory cytokine and growth factor release which perpetuates the vicious cycle of inflammation, lipid deposition and growth; ultimately forming an atherosclerotic plaque. The infiltration of monocytes through endothelial cells is accompanied by excessive ROS production through NADPH oxidase pathway, leading to further MMP activation [212].

It has been shown that the enhanced release of ROS from the foam cells during oxLDL phagocytosis increases MMP activity [213]. Endothelial dysfunction, one of the earliest events during atherogenesis, can be reversed in the rat by dietary supplementation of BH_4 that 're-couples' eNOS and enhances NO production [214]. ASAP (Antioxidant Supplementation in Atherosclerosis Prevention) have reported recently that long-term supplementation of vitamins C and E decreases the progression of carotid atherosclerosis [215].

Opposing the healing process of endothelial proliferation is apoptosis, which contributes to endothelial dysfunction [216,217]. Apoptosis in endothelial cells can be induced by a variety of factors, including hyperglycemia, oxLDL, TNF-α, and angiotensin II [218,219]. Ascorbate has been shown to prevent apoptosis due to inflammatory cytokines and oxidized LDL in cultured endothelial cells [217,219,220]. This is also evident *in vivo* as decreased release of microparticles derived from endothelial cells in subjects with congestive heart failure treated with vitamin C [221].

As noted previously, ascorbate stimulates all types of collagen synthesis, which allows proper folding into the triple helical collagen molecule that is then secreted to form the extracellular matrix, or to form part of the basement membrane with regard to type IV collagen. Lack of ascorbate thus prevents generation of mature type IV collagen by cultured endothelial cells [222]. Whereas deposition of any type of collagen may have the beneficial role in forming a "scar" and thus stabilizing a plaque in the vascular wall, lack of type IV collagen suggests dysfunctional or absent endothelial cells due to decreased proliferation or apoptosis [113]. Decreased collagen content translates to less stable atherosclerotic plaques, capable of rupture with associated thrombosis and infarction [223]. Increased collagen content and strength of the atherosclerotic plaque may also be part of the benefit afforded by lipid lowering [224] and statin [225] therapies.

The supplementation with ascorbic acid for 10 days was reported to reduce monocyte adhesiveness to endothelium in smokers [226]; however, another study showed no effect of ascorbic acid in monocyte adhesiveness [227], although supplementation in the latter lasted for a shorter period of time (2 hours). Also, there is evidence supporting a beneficial role of ascorbic acid in endothelium-dependent vasodilation, this way preventing endothelial dysfunction, as referred to in the Hypertension section. In rabbits, supplementation with ascorbic acid has been proved to prevent hypercholesterolemia-induced atherosclerosis [228].

Novel studies regarding the potentiation of vitamin E effects in association with vitamin C, as anti-atherogenic agents, are needed to understand the discrepancies between observational studies and randomized trials.

Antioxidant therapy is supposed to be rather effective in the early stages of atherosclerosis by preventing the oxidative lesion of endothelium and the LDL oxidation, than the clinical events in the advanced stages experienced by most patients participating in clinical trials. The protective effect shown by vitamin C and E supplementation in the prevention of immune atherosclerotic lesions occurring after cardiac transplant also supports this assumption [229,230]. In addition, several factors have been ignored by these studies, such as the genetic status of subjects, related with atherosclerosis-related polymorphisms [231-234]. This lack of benefit of antioxidants may reflect incomplete information on the actual role of oxidative stress, which should be considered as a necessary component of the enrolled patients, as antioxidants may have no effect in the absence of marked oxidative stress [103].

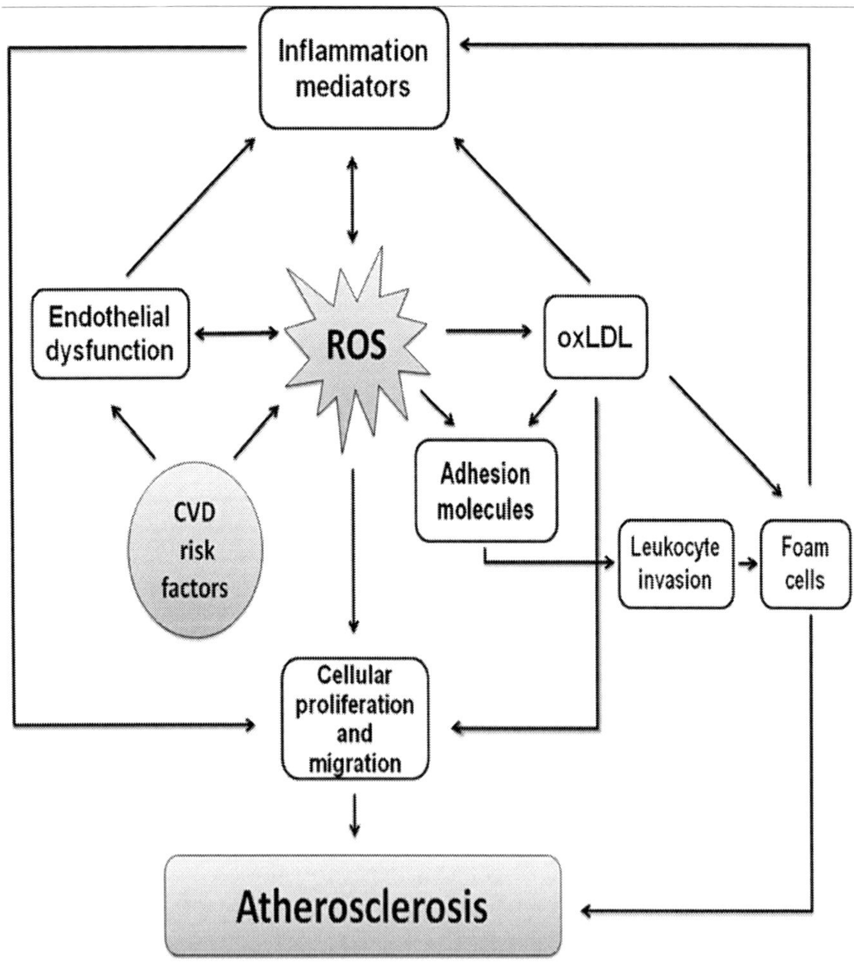

Figure 9. Scheme illustrating the hypothesis of the involvement of reactive oxygen species (ROS) in atherosclerosis. CVD, cardiovascular diseases; oxLDL, oxidized LDL. From: Molina V & Rodrigo R, 2009 [211], with permission.

III. Preeclampsia

Preeclampsia is a multisystem disorder of pregnancy whose cause remains largely unknown [103]. A large number of studies agree that preeclampsia is associated with a decrease in serum levels of ascorbic acid (vitamin C) and α-tocopherol (vitamin E) [235,236] as well as a decrease of other lipid soluble antioxidants such as coenzyme Q10 [237], carotenoids, and retinol [238].

Cumulated evidence points to a major role of oxidative stress as a factor underlying the mechanism of the development of the endothelial dysfunction accounting for the syndrome [239]. Therefore, the possibility aroused of a therapy aimed at oxidative stress reduction with antioxidant vitamins, based on the multiple biological properties of these agents in addition to prevention of lipid peroxidation [240]. These vitamins could play a key role in the modulation of enzymes involved in the vascular wall known to contribute to the pathophysiological mechanism of the clinical expression of preeclampsia. In all cell types of vascular cells, NADPH oxidase is the major source of superoxide anion radical, a key mediator in the development of systemic pathological processes such as impairment of endothelium-dependent vasodilation inflammation or increased platelet aggregation [241].

The activity of NADPH oxidase is directly downregulated by vitamins C and E [139], thereby contributing to counteract the development of these derangements in preeclampsia. These data are in agreement with previous studies demonstrating that both vitamins inhibit superoxide anion production in pig coronary artery [242]. In addition, in preparations of aorta from spontaneously hypertensive rats, it was found that vitamin C alone caused an enhancement of the activity of eNOS and NO generation [139], an effect expected to ameliorate the deleterious vascular consequences derived from endothelial dysfunction. The mechanisms whereby vitamins C and E may cause downregulation of NADPH oxidase and upregulation of eNOS are unclear, but it has been suggested that they may play an important role in the regulation of protein expression of the NADPH oxidase at the transcriptional or post-translational levels [243]. In addition, we should not discard the possibility that vitamins C and E directly influence the biological activity of the enzymes [241].

Another beneficial effect on endothelial cell function results from the ability of vitamins C and E to stimulate the activity of eNOS by increasing the intracellular availability of the eNOS cofactor tetrahydrobiopterin (BH_4) that would further increase NO synthesis [244,245], thus enhancing this enzyme activity. In addition, vitamin C treatment improves endothelial NO action, increases prostacyclin production, and lowers blood pressure in coronary patients [191,242,246].

Accordingly, several clinical trials have evaluated the effects of supplementation with vitamins C and E in pregnant women at high risk of preeclampsia, reporting some beneficial effect [247], not significant prevention [248,249], and lack of protection plus adverse effects [250]. The later study shows discrepancy with the previous data published by the same authors, who failed to give convincing explanation for this discrepancy. Indeed this study is focused on high-risk patients, within heterogeneous populations, including women with diabetes, chronic hypertension, renal disease, previous preeclampsia, antiphospholipid syndrome, obesity, and multiple births. Consequently, it could be expected that the preventive intervention might affect the disease subgroups differently. Another trial in nulliparous women showed that supplementation with vitamins C and E during pregnancy does not reduce the risk of preeclampsia in nulliparous women, the risk of intrauterine growth restriction, or the risk of death or other serious outcomes in their infants [251]. Unlike the study of Poston et al. [250], this study was performed with a homogeneous population, what make it a more acceptable trial. Several trials are being conducted in other subgroups of pregnant women, such as those having low risk or high risk, giving rise to different clinical outcomes resulting from vitamins C and E administration [241].

At present, the results of these studies have been mainly disappointing and controversial, but they should be interpreted with caution, as most of the data come from poor quality studies, due to methodological deficiencies related with both the characteristics of the patients recruited for the protocol and not enough early initiation of the treatment. In fact, most studies begin supplementation between 14 and 22 weeks of gestation, a time at which poor placentation could already have been established reaching the definite structural conformation of spiral arteries. Therefore, placental hypoperfusion is expected to occur due to lack of complete remodeling. It could be hypothesized that the derangement of placentation is a consequence of earlier events during gestation, based on the normal trophoblast invasion occurring in a way temporally and spatially unique that involves both degradative and adhesive interactions [252]. For successful invasion to occur, extravillous trophoblast has to perform a range of functions to proliferate, differentiate, adhere to and digest the extracellular matrix, move and interact with the maternal cells. Cytotrophoblast produces matrix metalloproteinases (MMP), which are responsible for remodeling of extracellular matrix, and specific adhesion molecules for both cell–cell interactions as well as cell– extracellular matrix interactions [ICAM-1 and vascular cell adhesion molecule-1 (VCAM-1)], thereby promoting invasion of maternal blood vessels to replace the endothelial cells and remodel vessel walls. Many of these adaptive changes appear to be disrupted in preeclampsia due to decreased degradative ability secondary to lower levels or cytokine inactivation of MMP-9 [253,254], or improper expression of adhesion molecules [255], all processes triggered by oxidative stress. Recently, placental oxidative stress has been attributed to increased expression of NADPH oxidase [256] and ET-1 [257] in the placenta, a process occurring very early during placental development, likely accounting for the impaired trophoblast migration and its consequences (Figure 11).

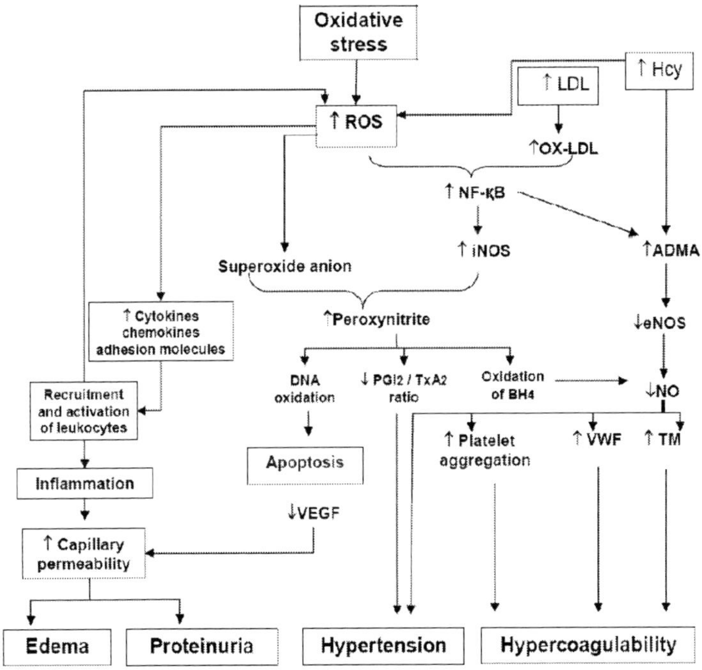

Figure 10. Diagram illustrating the proposed role of oxidative stress and the main contributory factors involving endothelial dysfunction, featuring clinical aspects of pre-eclampsia. ROS, reactive oxygen species; LDL, low density lipoproteins; Hcy, homocysteinemia; OX-LDL, oxidized LDL, NF-κB, nuclear factor kappa B; iNOS, inducible nitric oxide synthase; ADMA, asymmetric dimethyl-arginine; eNOS, endothelial nitric oxide synthase; VEGF, vascular endothelial growth factor; VWF, von Willebrand factor; TM, thrombomodulin; PGI_2, prostacyclin; TXA_2, thromoboxane A_2, BH_4, tetrahydrobiopterin. From: Parra M, 2009 [241], with permission.

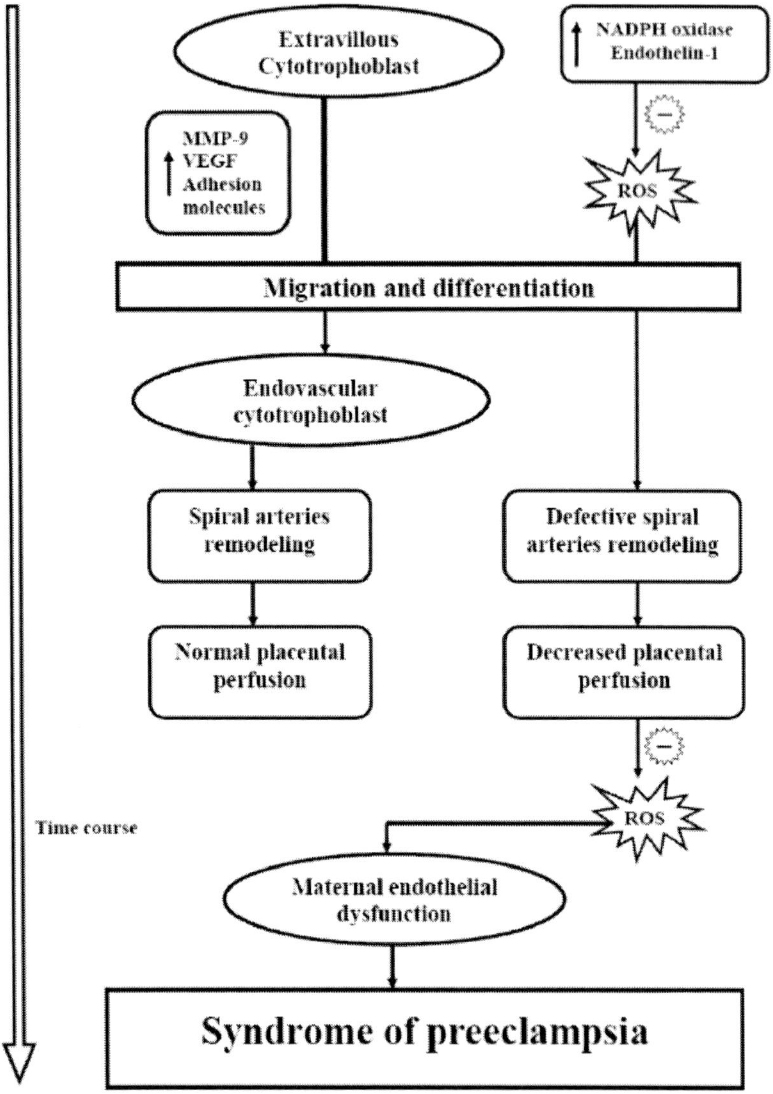

Figure 11. Hypothesis to explain the contribution of oxidative stress in the pathogenesis of the syndrome of pre-eclampsia. The counteracting effect of antioxidant vitamins C and E in two crucial stages of the process of placentation is indicated by the symbol (⊖). ROS, reactive oxygen species; MMP-9, matrix metaloproteinase-9; VEGF, vascular endothelial growth factor. From: Parra M, 2009 [241], with permission.

This view could explain the failure of the clinical trials to prevent the development of preeclampsia through later antioxidant therapy, a time of Doppler alterations consistent with diminished caliber of spiral arteries. It was claimed the importance of focusing in the knowledge of basic processes, with human studies stressing prediction markers combined with ancillary studies to help define the mechanisms, the safety, and efficacy of therapy, before applying expensive clinical trials [258]. Therefore, criteria other than Doppler consideration, such as earlier predictive test or clinical history, should be used to characterize the risk group enrolled to initiate antioxidant vitamins supplementation at the beginning of pregnancy to improve the maternal and fetal clinical outcome. Moreover, a recent epidemiological study of the intake of vitamins during pregnancy showed that preeclampsia could be prevented through a regular periconceptional use of vitamins [259], although this study was performed with uncertain doses of multivitamin supplements and not solely vitamins C and E.

The collective effort of clinicians, scientists, and patients will provide a definitive answer to whether the administration of vitamins C and E can prevent preeclampsia and if such an intervention would be safe.

IV. Post-Operative Atrial Fibrillation (POAF)

Oxidative stress has been strongly involved in the underlying mechanism of atrial fibrillation, particularly in the arrhythmia occurring in patients undergoing cardiac surgery with extracorporeal circulation (postoperative atrial fibrillation). The ischemia/reperfusion injury thus occurring in the myocardial tissue contributes to the development of tissue remodeling, thought to be responsible for the functional heart impairment. Consequently, structural changes due to the cardiac tissue biomolecules attack by ROS and/or reactive nitrogen species (RNS) could account for functional changes in ion channels, transporters, membrane conductance, cytosolic transduction signals, and other events, all associated with the occurrence of arrhythmic consequences (Figure 12). The lack of success and significant side effects of anti-arrhythmic drugs have given rise to attempts aimed to develop alternative novel pharmacologic treatments [260].

The effects of ascorbate administration in relation to atrial fibrillation (AF) have been tested under different contexts. One of the most paradigmatic studies involving ascorbate anti-arrhythmic properties was conducted to test not only the effects of vitamin C supplementation in POAF incidence, but also to assess the biochemical changes in oxidative and electric status after canine atrial pacing. In the first part, 43 patients subjected to coronary artery bypass were given 2 g of vitamin C the day before the surgery, followed by 500 mg until the fifth post-operative day. The POAF incidence in the ascorbate treated group was 16% v/s 35% in the control group. In the other part of the study, eleven dogs were subjected to rapid atrial pacing, which led to shortening of the effective refractory period (ERP), associated with accumulation of 3-nitrotyrosine, a peroxynitrite oxidative marker, and decreased levels of ascorbate compared with non paced controls. Ascorbate treatment attenuated the ERP shortening and diminished the 3-nitrotyrosine concentration found after atrial pacing [261]. This study showed, on the one hand that antioxidant vitamins could decrease the incidence of POAF, and on the other hand showed that this effect could be a reflection of a stabilization of the electrophysiological properties of the heart, that are impaired in individuals presenting this arrhythmia. It should be remembered that one of the mediators accounting for the shortening of the refractory period is superoxide (which leads to the cardiomyocytes calcium overloading), therefore it is plausible to occur an attenuation of the shortening ERP in presence of antioxidants [262].

A trial studied 44 patients subjected to electrical cardioversion of persistent AF, all received standard treatment, but one group received vitamin C during 7 days, while the other received only ordinary drugs. Within a week, AF recurred in 4.5% of the ascorbate treated group and in 36% of the control group [263]. In addition, antioxidant vitamins have been studied in the prevention of post-thrombolysis AF; comparing two groups subjected to therapeutic alteplase thrombolysis, one receiving antioxidant vitamins and the other placebo, the results showed that the first one developed AF after reperfusion in 6% while the placebo group presented the arrhythmia in 44% [264]. Post-thrombolysis AF is the gold standard example for ROS induced AF. Before the re-vascularization procedure, the heart tissue was experimenting high levels of hypoxia; whereas after the administration of the thrombolytic therapy (in this case alteplase), the heart suffered an acute restoration of blood and oxygen, which lead to calcium overloading of cardiomyocytes, activation of cell death pathways and production of high levels of ROS, phenomenon known as ischemia/reperfusion. Through all those mechanisms, electric properties of the heart were deregulated, and heart tissue was incapacitated to correctly conduct the electric impulses and therefore AF was observed [262].

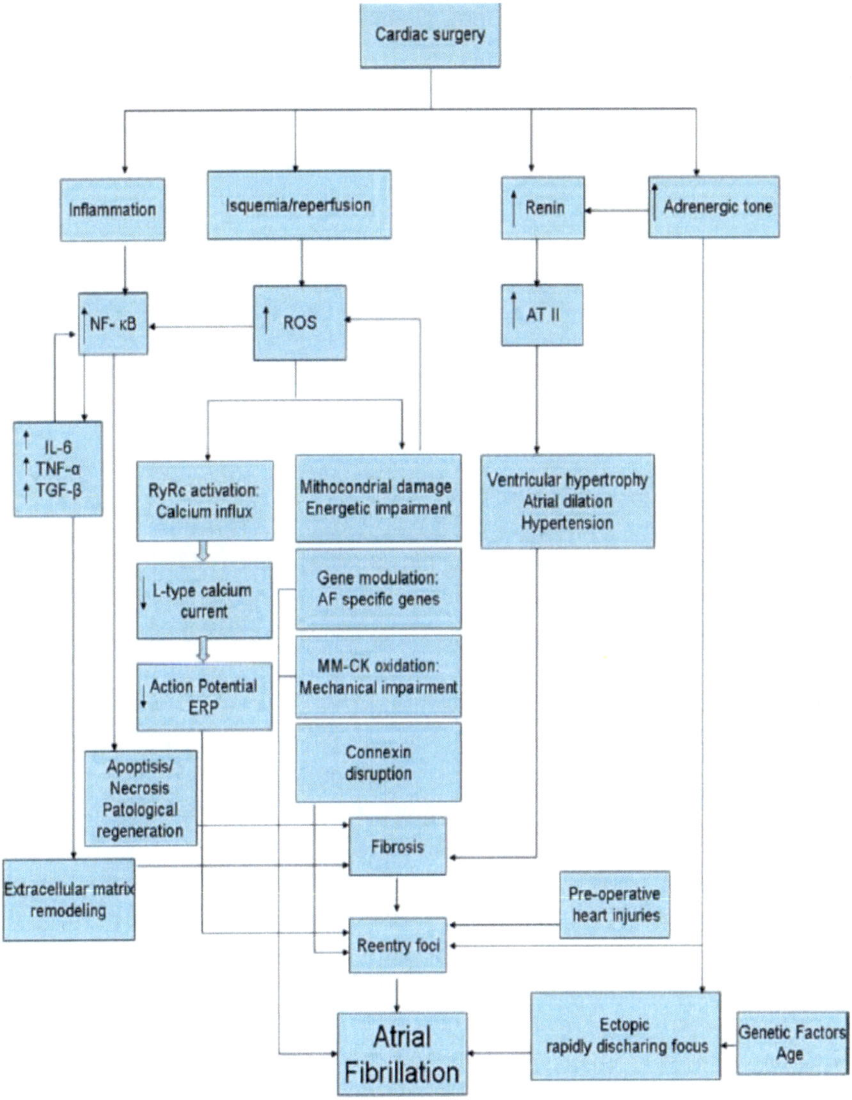

Figure 12. Schematic diagram illustrating a hypothesis based on the main contributory factors involved in the genesis and perpetuation of atrial fibrillation. AF, atrial fibrillation; NF-κB, nuclear factor kappaB; ROS, reactive oxygen species; AT II, angiotensin II; IL-6, interleukin-6; hsCRP, high sensitive C-reactive protein; RyRc, ryanodine receptor Ca^{2+} channel; ERP, effective refractory period; MM-CK, myofibrillar creatine kinase. Adapted from: Vinay J & Rodrigo R, 2009 [262], with permission.

Recently, it was shown that oral vitamin C in association with β-blockers was more effective in preventing POAF than β-blockers alone. This study consisted in 100 patients undergoing coronary artery bypass grafting, separated in a β-blockers group and a β-blockers/ascorbate group, which received 2 g of ascorbic acid on the night before the surgery and 2 g daily for 5 days after surgery. The POAF incidence was 4% in ascorbate group and 26% in the control group [265]. Consequently, antioxidant vitamins not only have shown favorable anti-arrhythmogenic results compared with non-vitamin patients, but also with patients receiving classical anti-AF drug treatment. This concept has major relevance, as the study for alternative therapeutic tools was originated due to the lack of effective and risk-free treatment for AF [262].

V. Metabolic Syndrome

The biochemical steps linking insulin resistance with the metabolic syndrome have not been completely clarified. Mounted experimental and clinical evidence indicates that oxidative stress is an attractive candidate for a central pathogenic role since it potentially explains the appearance of all risk factors and supports the clinical manifestations. Indeed, metabolic syndrome patients exhibit activation of biochemical pathways leading to increased delivery of ROS, decreased antioxidant protection and increased lipid peroxidation. The described associations between increased abdominal fat storage, liver steatosis and systemic oxidative stress, the diminished concentration of nitric oxide derivatives and antioxidant vitamins, and the endothelial oxidative damages observed in subjects with the metabolic syndrome support oxidative stress as the common second-level event in an unifying pathogenic view (Figure 13) [266].

In addition to the health effects of ascorbic acid as antioxidant, this vitamin could be involved in obesity-related mechanisms, for example, regulation of behavioural activity [267], lipolysis [268] and glucocorticoid release from the adrenal glands [269]. In hypertensive rats long term vitamin C administration significantly reduced systolic blood pressure and simultaneously reduced oxidative stress mediated by NAD(P)H oxidase activation [270]. Vitamin C has beneficial effects not only on blood pressure but also on endothelial function in hypertensive and diabetic patients [271]. Vitamin C administration ameliorates hyperglycemia and glycosylation in diabetic-obese rodents [272] and inhibits the activation of inflammatory response mediated by nuclear factor-kappa B [273]. Vitamin C is a soluble compound and it prevents protein and lipid oxidation in the extracellular environment [274]. In vivo studies confirmed that vitamin C administration improves arterial vasodilatation by increasing NO production [139].

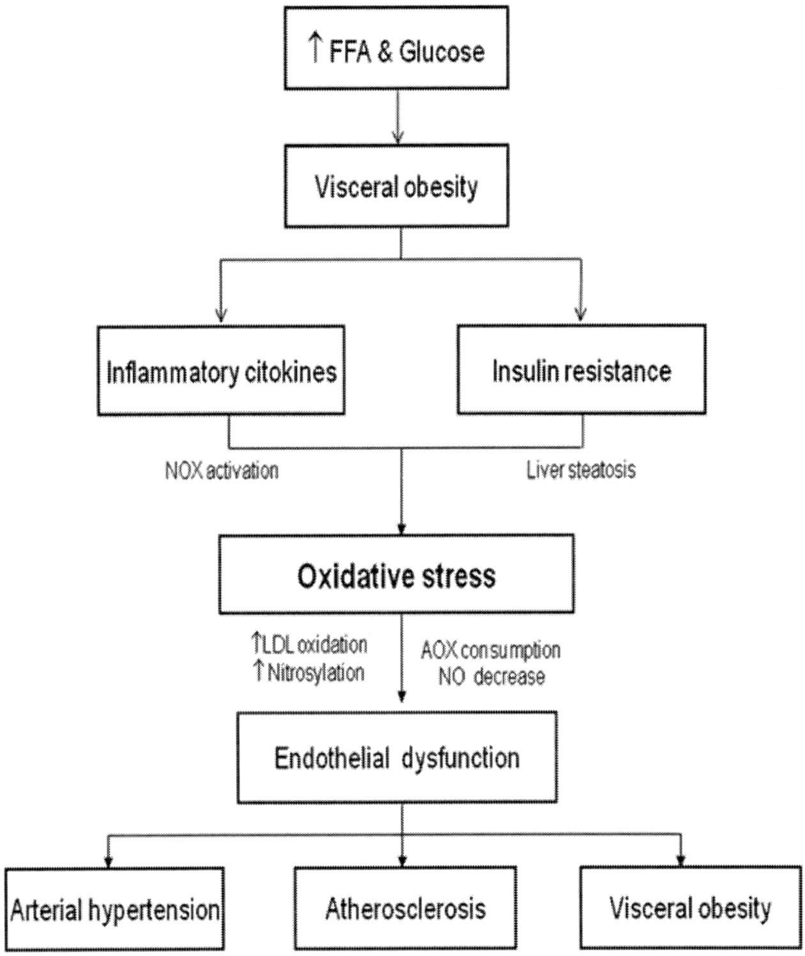

Figure 13. ROS generation and consequent oxidative stress as a "second-level" event causing metabolic syndrome-associated. FFA: Free fatty acids; NOX: NADPH oxidase; LDL: Low-density , lipoprotein; AOX: Antioxidant defenses; NO: nitric oxide. From: Castillo, 2009a [266], with permission.

VI. Diabetes Mellitus

Insulin resistance is a cardinal feature of type 2 diabetes. Recently, it has been proposed that ROS have a causal role in multiple forms of insulin resistance [275]. Elevation of glycemia in diabetic patients may lead to the autooxidation of glucose, glycation of proteins, and the activation of polyol metabolism (Figure 14). These changes accelerate the generation of reactive oxygen species and increase oxidative modification of lipids, DNA, and proteins in various tissues. Thus, oxidative stress occurring in this setting may play an important role in the development of the chronic complications of diabetes, such as nephropathy, neuropathy, and lens cataracts [276].

Diabetic patients show, during the postprandial period, an increase in MDA plasma levels and a decrease in sulphydryl groups, α-tocopherol and total radical-trapping antioxidant parameter [277]. The latter observation might be related to the significantly lower levels of ascorbic acid and urate observed in diabetic patients, although dietary intake should be considered when explaining changes in plasma antioxidant levels [278].

There exists evidence that the over expression of antioxidants such as Cu/Zn superoxide dismutase [279], catalase [280], thioredoxin [281], and metallothionein [282] targeted at β-cells counteracts the development of type 1 diabetes. Since the pancreas has been shown to have low levels of the antioxidant enzymes superoxide dismutase and catalase [283], these findings suggest that oxidative stress plays a key role in the pathogenesis of diabetes [284]. Indeed, peroxynitrite, which is the product of the reaction between NO and superoxide, induced by inflammatory cytokines such as interleukin-1β, TNF-α, and interferon-γ are considered to be crucial mediators of β-cell death [285,286].

This is supported by several studies showing that pretreatment with antioxidants before the injection of streptozotocin (STZ, a compound selectively toxic to pancreatic beta cells) attenuates the development of hyperglycemia and insulitis in the multiple low-dose streptozotocin models [287-289]. Experimental models in STZ-treated rats have been used to assess the effect of short-term antioxidant therapy based on oral vitamins C and E administration, with similar antioxidant response [290,291].

In the case of vitamin C, the use for attenuating oxidative injury might become a useful adjunct to prevent albuminuria and renal sclerosis in rat diabetic nephropathy [292]. It was demonstrated that ascorbic acid directly modulates contractile responses of diabetic rat aortas, likely through mechanisms in part dependent of preservation of endothelium-derived NO

[293]. In this point, vitamin C may act as a direct ROS scavenger in endothelium; resulting in increased availability of the eNOS cofactor tetrahydrobiopterin, thereby enhancing eNOS activity [294].

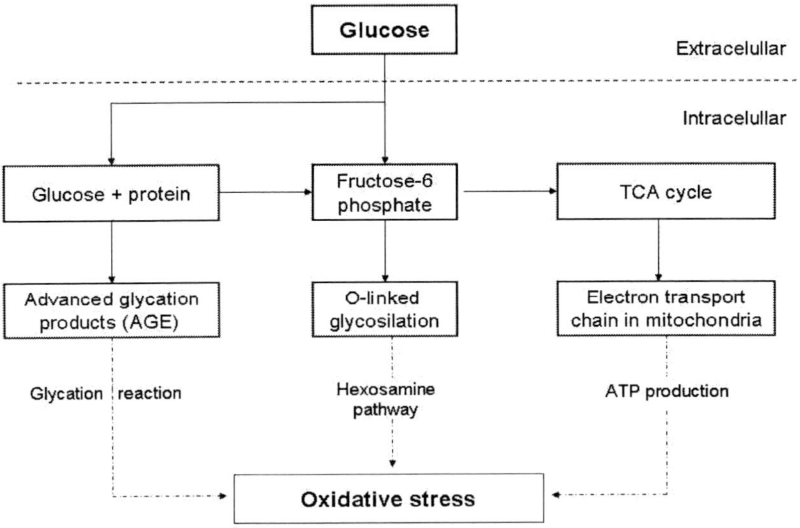

Figure 14. Sources of cellular ROS in chronic hyperglycemia TCA, Tricarboxylic acid. From: Castillo, 2009b [276], with permission.

VII. Non-Alcoholic Steatohepatitis (NASH)

Oxidative stress caused by increased ROS plays an important role in the pathogenesis of NASH [295].

The sole clinical trial testing the effect of vitamin C in NASH patients is difficult to, as it has been assayed in combination with vitamin E [296]. Nevertheless, vitamin C, in addition to its direct free radical scavenging abilities, has the property to regenerate oxidized vitamin E and glutathione to the reduced active forms [297].

Some animal studies have shown that vitamin C is able to improve liver antioxidant defenses [298] and others showed that it can prevent liver induced oxidative damage [299]. Thus, it is reasonable to think that vitamin C therapy could improve NASH [295].

VIII. Ischemia-Reperfusion

ROS generated from metabolic processes are normally quenched by antioxidants that are part of physiological cellular defense mechanisms. In disease states such as sudden hypoxia, however, overproduction of ROS and consumption of antioxidants result in oxidative cellular damage [300]. Rapid restoration of blood flow increases the level of tissue oxygenation, but there is a second burst of ROS generation that leads to the syndrome of reperfusion injury [301]. ROS-mediated cell death occurs in cells exposed to hypoxia and hypoxia/reoxygenation both *in vitro* and *in vivo* [302,303].

In ischemia–reperfusion, the enzyme xanthine oxidase catalyses the formation of uric acid with the co-production of superoxide. Superoxide release results in the recruitment and activation of neutrophils and their adherence to endothelial cells, which stimulates the formation of xanthine oxidase in the endothelium, with further superoxide production [103]. Although the role of xanthine oxidase in oxidative damage by ischemia–reperfusion remains controversial, this enzyme appears to be an important source of ROS production in this pathophysiological condition [304,305]. Accordingly, allopurinol, a xanthine oxidase inhibitor, has been demonstrated that blocks the superoxide production in ischemia–reperfusion settings involving organs such as heart [306], liver [304], kidney [307], and small intestine [308].

Oxidation of DNA and proteins may take place, along with membrane damage, because of lipid peroxidation, leading to alterations in membrane permeability, modification of protein structure and functional changes [309]. Oxidative damage to the mitochondrial membrane can also occur, resulting in membrane depolarization and the uncoupling of oxidative phosphorylation, with altered cellular respiration [310]. This can ultimately lead to mitochondrial damage, with release of cytochrome c, activation of caspases and apoptosis [311].

IX. Acute Myocardial Infarction

Acute myocardial infarction is an important ischemic heart disease and a leading cause of morbidity and mortality worldwide [302]. It is well recognized that myocardial infarction is a complex phenomenon affecting the mechanical, electrical, structural and biochemical properties of the heart [312].

Despite of this complexity, impressive recent progress has been achieved in advancing our understanding of cellular processes and mechanistic bases underlying cardiac dysfunction associated with myocardial infarction and most importantly, in applying this knowledge to therapeutic interventions [313].

Myocardial ischemic injury is mediated in part by ROS produced during the ischemic process and exacerbated by reperfusion [302,314]. ROS cause oxidation of proteins, nucleic acids, and lipids and can affect critical signal transduction pathways, resulting in alterations of cardiac function, cellular injury, and death [315-317]. In the heart, ROS-induced abnormalities can include cytotoxicity, cardiac stunning, arrhythmias, alterations of Ca^{2+} homeostasis, and intracellular ATP depletion [302,314]. Despite evidence that implicates ROS in cardiac dysfunction, the molecular mechanisms by which ROS induce cardiac damage remains largely unknown and it is uncertain to what extent ROS are directly involved in the myocardial necrosis that characterizes a myocardial infarct.

Only one randomized, double-blind, placebo controlled study [318] has been published using vitamin C (1000 mg/12 h infusion) followed by 1200 mg/24 h orally and vitamin E (600 mg/24 h) for 30 days. Even though this study has significant methodological deficiencies, it suggests that supplementation with these antioxidant vitamins seems to positively influence the clinical outcome of patients with AMI, in terms of composite of in-hospital cardiac mortality, non-fatal new myocardial infarction, ventricular tachicardia/ventricular fibrillation/asystole or shock/pulmonary edema.

Furthermore, in a retrospective analysis of the aforementioned data [319], it has been found a significant reduction in 30-day cardiac mortality in diabetic patients treated with vitamins C and E. In patients without diabetes, the administration of vitamins had no such effect on cardiac mortality. This result on diabetic patients with AMI seems to be particularly reasonable because of the increased ROS formation in these patients, already reviewed on the diabetes mellitus section.

Other studies [320,321] have published positive results for vitamin C combined with other vitamins or a diuretic. Therefore methodological limitations demand cautious interpretation of the results [318]. The issue of vitamin C protection in human AMI remains open. It should be noted that although some beneficial effect derived from the biological properties of antioxidant vitamins could be expected in the patients subjected to these protocols. However, the most important function to abrogate oxidative stress-dependent processes cannot be achieved by the vitamin C doses used in any of these studies. Indeed, it is necessary to reach plasma levels of ascorbate about

10 mmol/L to prevent the chemical reaction of NO and superoxide anion, otherwise resulting in a highly peroxidant pathway.

Regarding rats, in a study published by Guaiquil et al. [322] cardiomyocytes in culture incubated with DHA could accumulate intracellular concentrations of ascorbate as high as 39 mmol/L. *In vivo*, the ascorbate content in hearts was six to eight times higher in DHA-treated animals than in those untreated or treated with ascorbate. DHA administration before or after coronary ligation resulted in an increased concentration of ascorbate in the heart from a basal 0.4 μmol/L to 3 and 1 mmol/L, respectively. Loading the cardiomyocytes with ascorbate by DHA treatment resulted in a significant degree of protection from cell death due to hypoxia or hypoxia/ reoxygenation. Myocardial protection in the *in vivo* coronary ligation model was substantial. DHA treatment before coronary ligation consistently reduced the area of infarcted myocardium by more than 60%. Importantly, they observed reduction of infarct size when DHA was administered intraperitoneally 1 h postligation or after 2 h when DHA was given intravenously. Surprisingly, pretreatment with ascorbate, however, provided no significant myocardial protection.

As an explanation for this fact, both rats and humans express the SVCT2 protein in the heart [323,324], so the issue turns to capacities of the transport mechanisms. As DHA moves energetically driven trough a facilitated transport mechanism, high plasma concentrations of this compound would result in acquiring of DHA by the GLUTs and reduction to ascorbate. On the other hand, ascorbate energy requiring transporters will be placed in a setting of reduced Na^+ driving force due to energy starvation and cell sodium overloading, therefore decreasing the chance of ascorbate to be transported into the cell.

During reoxygenation, normal metabolic processes are restored and a second burst of ROS is produced which may increase cellular damage. Characterization of apoptosis in cells subjected to hypoxia/ reoxygenation showed upregulation of the pro-apoptotic protein Bax, release of cytochrome c into the cytoplasm, and activation of caspase-3 [322]. In these cells, DHA treatment inhibited cell death and the activation of proapoptotic proteins, and resulted in upregulation of the antiapoptotic proteins Bcl-2 and Bcl-xl. The exact mechanisms by which vitamin C protects the cardiomyocytes and myocardial tissue are uncertain, however, ROS generation in hypoxic cardiomyocytes was markedly inhibited in cells preloaded with vitamin C.

Another study in rats using an isoproterenol AMI model [325], showed a reduction in the degenerative changes of the myocardial tissue. Vitamin C was able to exert anti-oxidant activity as depicted by suppressing iNOS synthesis on heart damaged cells. These rats received vitamin C, 150 mg/kg, orally for seven consecutive days. At days 5 and 6 the rats were submitted to acute administration of isoproterenol 150 mg/kg, subcutaneous.

In conclusion, vitamin C seems to have a helpful effect by means of tackling the pathophysiological mechanisms of AMI. Previous studies have reported sub-optimal results in humans, likely due to the achievement of plasma ascorbate concentration lower than that required to prevent oxidative stress-derived processes. Further investigation in humans will be necessary to elucidate this hypothesis.

X. Acute Cerebrovascular Attack

Perhaps the most dramatic acute oxidant stress in the CNS is the ischemia–reperfusion injury that occurs with ischemic stroke. Ischemia initially depletes intracellular ascorbate [326] and GSH [327] in the brain. If reperfusion with oxygen-rich blood occurs, the ROS generated by abnormal mitochondrial metabolism will extend tissue damage to areas with decreased oxidant defenses [328].

Parenteral ascorbate injections decreased infarct size in both primate and rodent models of middle cerebral artery ischemia–reperfusion. When monkeys were given 1 g/day of ascorbate parenterally for 6 days before middle cerebral artery occlusion, brain infarct size was decreased by 50% in the ascorbate-treated group compared to the control group not treated with ascorbate [329]. Ascorbate was measured in the basal ganglia of these animals and was found to increase 50% above levels in the treated compared to the untreated monkeys [329]. Thus, relatively modest increases in brain ascorbate content due to several days of parenteral administration were associated with neuroprotection against ischemia–reperfusion injury. In another primate study, high-dose ascorbate (500 mg/kg up to 2 g) was administered into the middle cerebral artery just before occlusion, which was maintained for 4 hours. At 24 hours after reperfusion, the mean infarct size in ascorbate-treated monkeys was only one third of that in untreated controls. This dramatic decrease in infarct size with acute dosing was surprising, given that ascorbate normally enters the CNS slowly through the choroid plexus. Even though glia may not normally express the SVCT2, oxidant stress due to ischemia– reperfusion injury has been shown to increase SVCT2 mRNA expression in both neurons and glia [330].

In a subsequent study in mice with middle cerebral artery occlusion, high-dose DHA given by intraluminal infusion injection just before, 15 minutes after, or 3 hours after occlusion markedly decreased infarct volume, mortality, and neurological deficits in mice [331]. Protection by DHA infusion was observed in both ischemia alone and ischemia–reperfusion models. A subsequent study by the same group [332] replicated the initial results in mice and further showed that postischemic DHA infusion prevented the 50% decrease in brain ascorbate and also largely prevented the increase in lipid peroxidation due to ischemia–reperfusion injury. Why ascorbate infusion decreased lesion size in the primate study but not in the mouse studies is unclear, but it could relate to breakdown of the blood–brain barrier in ischemic regions, thus allowing entry of both ascorbate and DHA, or to differences in the ability of ascorbate to gain access to the CNS in the two species. That is, the loss of the ability to synthesize ascorbate may have favored development of alternate routes or of more rapid transit of ascorbate into the CNS in primates [53].

XI. Cancer

Like many redox molecules, ascorbate can act either as a pro-oxidant or a reducing (i.e., anti-oxidant) agent depending on the redox status of the cell and its environment, as well as the concentration of ascorbate at the specific time [300,333]. Accordingly, ascorbate can generate hydrogen peroxide upon oxidation in biological systems. This action can be enhanced by divalent cations such as iron and copper. Hydrogen peroxide may further generate additional reactive species and secondary products of oxidation.

In general, the cytotoxicity induced by ascorbate seems to be primarily mediated by hydrogen peroxide generated be the cells is proportionally dependent on the ascorbate concentration and inhibited by serum (i.e., serum contains antioxidants). Hydrogen peroxide is most likely generated intracellularly during ascorbate metabolic oxidation to dehydroascorbate. The hydrogen peroxide reduces cellular levels of thiols and can initiate membrane lipid peroxidation [333]. Also, it should be emphasized that ascorbate cytotoxic action can be enhanced by the inclusion of synergistic substances (e.g., futile redox cycling quinones) [27].

The vitamin C free radical species, ascorbyl radical, is detectable in animals only when they receive intravenous vitamin C equivalent to a 10-g dose in humans [334]. It has been proposed that detectable ascorbyl radical forms only when human plasma concentrations are greater than 1000 μmol/L and that either the radical itself or its unpaired electron induces oxidative damage that can be repaired by normal but not cancer cells [34].

Several studies in the literature show that the urinary excretion of ascorbate is reduced in patients with cancer when compared to healthy individuals. Spellberg and Keeton have reported that after continued daily oral administration of 400 mg of vitamin C, healthy persons excreted 56% to 80% of intake, whereas cancer patients excreted only 34 to 48% [335]. Likewise, Bodansky reported a daily urinary excretion of vitamin C in two cancer patients that ranged from 5 to 10% of the intake [336]. This decreased percentage of ascorbate excretion in urine after daily oral intake under a controlled metabolic regimen reflects a higher consumption of ascorbate by cancerous patients. This is probably related to certain metabolic differences between patients and healthy individuals [27]. Studies by Holmes and co-workers indicated that healthy persons excrete about 30 to 50% of a daily intake of about 100 mg ascorbate and even higher percentages at greater intakes [337,338]. Certainly, several studies show that the urinary excretion of ascorbate is less in cancer patients than in normal people [335,336].

Cancer cells can absorb high levels of ascorbate (that is, at millimolar range) and unlike normal tissues their disturbed metabolism produces redox cycling and Fenton-type, Fe^{2+}-mediated, free radicals. Since tumor cells are often catalase deficient, they are more sensitive to cytotoxic levels of hydrogen peroxide than normal cells [339]. The preferential ascorbate accumulation /replenish process in the store tissues is evident in tumors, which may provide a therapeutic advantage, as these high ascorbate amounts may be enough for its cytotoxic action. In addition, damaged tissues like cancer cells are highly demanding compartments that can absorb high levels of ascorbate (at millimolar range). Consequently, the consumption of higher ascorbate amounts by these tissues accounts for most of the systemic ascorbate in excess. Published studies show that intravenous ascorbate dosing schemes can be properly used in order to achieve plasma levels equivalent to those reported as necessary to kill tumor cells [340-342].

Indeed, *in vitro* evidence showed that vitamin C killed cancer cells at extracellular concentrations higher than 1000 μmol/L [343,344], and its clinical use by some practitioners continues [38].

It has been reported cytotoxicity greater than 97% for the serum samples taken at 35, 65, and 95 minutes after the beginning of IV injection of vitamin C. During those periods the serum concentration was greater than 400 mg/dL. After that time the toxicity decreased. The last sample taken (vitamin C concentration 213 mg/dL) resulted in 64% inhibition compared to the controls [345].

Despite poor rationale, vitamin C in gram doses was proposed as an anticancer agent decades ago [346]. Unblinded studies with retrospective or nonrandom controls reported clinical benefit from oral and intravenous vitamin C administered to patients with terminal cancer at a dosage of 10 g daily [155,347,348]. Placebo-controlled trials in patients with cancer reported no benefit from oral vitamin C at a dosage of 10 g daily [349,350], and vitamin C treatment was judged ineffective [351]. These results cannot be compared due to the huge differences in ascorbate pharmacokinetics through oral or intravenous dosing, already stated in the Pharmacokinetics section.

Case series published by Cameron, Campbell, and Pauling [155,347,348] have been controversial. In these series, several hundred patients with terminal cancer treated with 10 g of vitamin C intravenously for 10 days and then 10 g orally indefinitely were compared with more than 1000 retrospective and prospective controls. Patients treated with vitamin C survived 150 to 300 days longer than controls [155,347,348]. Other researchers reported benefit consisting of increased survival, improved well-being, and reduced pain [155]. All of these studies were uncontrolled, and factors unrelated to intervention may have affected outcome.

However, consumption of fruits and vegetables, which contain vitamin C, is beneficial for unknown reasons [29,352]. On the basis of current knowledge and the pharmacokinetics presented here, physicians should advise their patients to consume fruits and vegetables, not vitamin C supplements, to obtain potential benefits [38].

XII. Glaucoma

The involvement of ROS in the pathogenesis of glaucoma is supported by various experimental findings, including: (i) resistance to aqueous humor outflow is increased by hydrogen peroxide by inducing trabecular meshwork (TM) degeneration; (ii) TM possesses remarkable antioxidant potential, mainly explained by superoxide dismutase and catalase activities and glutathione pathways, all that is found decreased in glaucoma patients; and (iii) intraocular-pressure increase and severity of visual-field defects in glaucoma patients paralleled by the amount of oxidative damage of DNA affecting TM [353].

Ascorbate protects low-density lipoprotein cholesterol from oxidative damage and reduces platelet aggregation [354]. By enhancing NO synthase activity, vitamin C is potentially important in lowering blood pressure [244]. The administration of ascorbic acid appears to have a transient hypotonic effect on intraocular pressure in normal eyes [353]. Its effect on glaucomatous eyes is not well defined particularly in the case of the rabbit model [355]. Osmolarity is suggested as a possible hypotensive mechanism and a differential fluid transport rate between the blood and the aqueous humor for the different genotypes is suggested as a possible mechanism for the difference in duration [356]. With respect to doses, the weight of available evidence supports the role of vitamin C in prevention of lens opacities, and the adverse reactions reported to have occurred above the dosage of 1000 mg per day [357].

XIII. Age Related Macular Degeneration

Vitamin C supplements combined with other antioxidant vitamins and minerals have been found to slow down the progression of advanced age-related macular degeneration and loss of visual acuity in people with signs of this disease [358,359].

Chapter V

Side Effects

The routine dietary supplementation with antioxidant vitamins has been used to delay the onset of chronic human diseases. Nevertheless, their beneficial effects have been questioned and, in some cases, reported harmful [360,361]. The potential toxicity of excessive doses of supplemental vitamin C relates to intraintestinal events and to the effects of metabolites in the urinary system [103].

Intakes of 2–3 g/day of vitamin C produce unpleasant diarrhea from the osmotic effects of the unabsorbed vitamin in the intestinal lumen in most healthy people [362]. Gastrointestinal disturbances can occur after ingestion of as little as 1 g because approximately half of this amount would not be absorbed at this dose [42].

Oxalate is an end-product of ascorbate catabolism and plays an important role in kidney stone formation. Excessive daily amounts of vitamin C produce hyperoxaluria. In four volunteers who received vitamin C in doses ranging from 5 to 10 g/day, mean urinary oxalate excretion approximately doubled from 50 to 87 mg/day (range, 60–126 mg/day) [363]. However, the risk of oxalate stone formation may become significant at high intakes of vitamin C (>1 g/day) [364], particularly in subjects with high amounts of urinary calcium [363]. The association between ascorbate supplementation and increased risk of kidney stone formation remains a matter of controversy [365].

In patients with renal failure, vitamin C is retained and converted to insoluble oxalate, which can accumulate in various organs. In a case report, the administration of vitamin C (self-medication 2 g/day for 3 years while in dialysis) led to the development of renal failure after kidney transplantation, due to the widespread deposition of calcium oxalate crystals [366]. Therefore, high-dose vitamin C therapy should be avoided in patients with renal failure or renal insufficiency, and in patients undergoing dialysis [25,367,368].

Vitamin C may precipitate haemolysis in some people, including those with glucose-6-phosphate dehydrogenase deficiency [369], paroxysmal nocturnal haemaglobinuria [370], or other conditions where increased risk of red cell haemolysis may occur or where protection against the removal of the products of iron metabolism may be impaired, as in people with the haptoglobin Hp2-2 phenotype [371]. Of these, only the haptoglobin Hp2-2 condition was associated with abnormal vitamin C metabolism (lower plasma ascorbate than expected) and only in cases where intake of vitamin C was provided mainly from dietary sources [7].

The studies in which brain ascorbate was measured clearly support the notion that increases in brain ascorbate concentrations can be beneficial in ischemia or ischemia–reperfusion models of stroke. They also allay to some extent the concern raised by a human study of acute parenteral ascorbate prophylaxis before ischemia–reperfusion related to abdominal vascular surgery [372]. In that study intravenous ascorbate infusion (2 g given 2 hours before ischemia was induced) increased tissue release of ROS, possibly owing to a Fenton-type reaction of ascorbate with free iron in ischemic areas. This was thought in turn to account for the increased generation of lipid peroxides and inflammatory cytokines observed. That opposite results were seen after middle cerebral artery occlusion suggests that ascorbate did not encounter significant amounts of free iron in the brain. Such iron would probably be outside living cells, where it would encounter only nonreactive DHA in the DHA infusion studies. This DHA would be taken up and to ascorbate intracellularly, where it would not have exposure to free iron [53].

In ischemia-reperfusion models, high DHA doses may be toxic to some cell types, such as insulin-secreting cells of islets [373]. In contrast to the results with DHA, no effects were observed for comparable injections of ascorbate [53].

However, a robust database shows that dietary supplements of these vitamins are safe for the general population [374].

Chapter VI

Conclusions

Vitamin C is a potent water-soluble antioxidant synthesized from glucose in most mammalian species, but not in humans. Nevertheless, ascorbate is found in many fruits and vegetables. At the same time, the wide consumption of orange juice should be encouraged, given that little amounts of this natural juice will fulfill the needs of every healthy person.

At present, vitamin C deficiency states are extremely uncommon in humans as a well-balanced diet provides adequate amounts of this vitamin. The recommended dietary allowance must be consulted before assessing individual requirements, for one recommendation cannot fit all categories of patients.

Fortunately, scurvy seems a disease of old sailors. Nevertheless, the socio-economical situations of its appearance in the modern world should not be forgotten, i.e.: famine, war, regularity of fruit and vegetable consumption, cultural preferences and cost.

Concerning the pharmacokinetic properties of vitamin C, the intestinal absorption encompases a 70-90% range. Besides bioavailability of vitamin C, its physiologically efficient renal-tubular reabsorption mechanism preserves vitamin C at steady-state plasma concentrations from 70 to 85 µmol/L. Peak values do not exceed 220 µmol/L, even after maximum oral administration of 3 g 6 times daily (18 g total), saturating the body. Even so, the tissues become saturated up to a whole-body content of ascorbate of about 20 mg/kg body weight and no further. Ascorbate has a half-life of about 30 minutes when plasma levels are by 70 µmol/L. Moreover, an elevated level of ascorbate in the intestinal lumen leads to down-regulation of the transporters in enterocytes, which underlies the limitations of oral supplementation.

By contrast, intravenous vitamin C may produce plasma concentrations as high as 15000 μmol/L.

Sodium- and energy-dependent transport of vitamin C is necessary to achieve a concentration gradient from blood or the interstitium into cells. In addition to ascorbate uptake through the SVCT proteins, DHA can enter and leave cells by facilitated diffusion on the ubiquitous glucose transporters of the GLUT family. For these reasons, some cell types accumulate ascorbate amounts above the actual plasma levels. This is also enhanced by multiple intracellular recycling mechanisms helping to maintain high intracellular ascorbate levels.

As a pleitropic molecule, vitamin C has various functions. As an antioxidant it counteracts and prevents the oxidation of lipids, proteins and DNA, subsequently protecting their structure and biological function. Ascorbate in aqueous compartments can also recycle α-tocopherol. As an enzymatic cofactor vitamin C acts as an electron donor for eight human enzymes facilitating collagen synthesis and maturation. Vast effects on brain neurotransmission, regarding dopamine- and glutamate-mediated neurotransmission, norepinephrine biosynthesis, acetylcholine and catecholamine release, neuropeptide amidation and release and myelin sheath synthesis. Blood pressure modulation can also be dependent on the activity of eNOS, whose function is linked to availability of BH_4, a cofactor preserved by vitamin C in its reduced state.

The clinical use of antioxidant vitamins has gained considerable interest during the last decades, since they could account for an effective protection against many diseases related with oxidative stress. However, their efficacy remains controversial in the light of some recent clinical trials and meta-analyses. Many reasons in relation to vitamin C can account for these inconsistencies.

In the first place, and as thoroughly reviewed on this chapter, vitamin C oral supplements cannot attain ascorbate millimolar concentrations. Therefore, lack of benefit should be expected from the superoxide scavenging properties of ascorbate oral supplementation protocols.

Second, some diseases, such as preeclampsia, lack a detailed pathophysiology particularly in terms of timings. On the other hand, there may be years-length pathophysiological cumulative abnormalities, i.e.: atherosclerosis. This leads to the "too little, too late" issue, for antioxidants can certainly not act retrospectively.

And third, most diseases affecting humans are multi-causal. Thus, appropriate antioxidant supplementation with vitamin C may be able to tackle only one cornerstone involved in the development of such disease.

Despite the aforementioned, promising results have been achieved in hypertension, post-operatory atrial fibrillation and acute myocardial infarction, among others.

A joint effort between basic researchers and clinicians must be made in order to fully assess the contribution of oxidative stress in the pathophysiology of disease. This will provide the necessary information to design goal directed strategies to supplement patients which should result in benefit for the patients, because the side effects seem to be minimal if any, compared to the large store of drugs and their countless side effects.

References

[1] James Lind: A *Treatise of the Scurvy,* 1753.

[2] Kramer JGH: Medicina castrensis. Wien, 1739.

[3] Mandl J, Szarka A, Bánhegyi G. Vitamin C: update on physiology and pharmacology. *Br. J. Pharmacol.* 2009;157:1097–1110

[4] Stone I. The Healing Factor: Vitamin C against Disease. Putnam Pub Group, New York. 1974.

[5] Mackenzie B, Illing A, Hediger M. Transport model of the human Na+-coupled L-ascorbic acid (vitamin C) transporter SVCT1. *Am. J. Physiol. Cell Physiol.* 2008;294:451-459.

[6] Haytowitz D.B. Information from USDA's Nutrient Data Bank. *J. Nutr.* 1995;125 1952–1955.

[7] World Health Organization, Food and Agricultural Organization of the United Nations. Vitamin and mineral requirements in human nutrition, 2nd edition. China, WHO/FAO, 2004.

[8] Pisoschi AM, Danet AF, Kalinowski S. Ascorbic Acid determination in commercial fruit juice samples by cyclic voltammetry. *J. Autom. Methods Manag. Chem.* 2008;2008:937651.

[9] Olmedo JM, Yiannias JA, Windgassen EB, Gornet MK. Scurvy: a disease almost forgotten. *Int. J. Dermatol.* 2006;45:909–913.

[10] Brigelius-Flohé R, Roob JM, Tiran B, Wuga S. The effect of age on vitamin E status, metabolism, and function: metabolism as assessed by labeled tocopherols. *N. Y. Acad. Sci.* 2004;1031:40–43.

[11] Berger M. Vitamin C Requirements in Parenteral Nutrition. *Gastroenterology.* 2009;137:S70 S78

[12] Food and Nutrition Board. Dietary reference intakes: applications in dietary assessment. Washington, DC, National Academy Press, 2001.

[13] Panel on Dietary Antioxidants and Related Compounds, Subcommittee on Upper Reference Levels of Nutrients, Subcommittee on Interpretation and Uses of DRIs, Standing Committee on the Scientific Evaluation of Dietary Reference Intakes, Food and Nutrition Board, Institute of Medicine. Dietary Reference Intakes for Vitamin C, Vitamin E, Selenium, and Carotenoids. 1st edition. Washington, DC, National Academy Press. 2000.

[14] Jennings PE, Chirico S, Jones AF, Lunec J, Barnett AH. Vitamin C metabolites and microangiography in diabetes mellitus. *Diabetes Res.* 1987;6:151–154.

[15] Thurnham DI. beta-Carotene, are we misreading the signals in risk groups? Some analogies with vitamin C. *Proc. Nutr. Soc.* 1994;53:557–569.

[16] Faruque MO, Khan MR, Rahman MM, Ahmed F. Relationship between smoking and antioxidant status. *Br. J. Nutr.* 1995;73:625–632.

[17] Finch S, Smithers G, Doyle W, Lowe C, Bates CJ, Prentice A, Clarke PC. National diet and nutrition survey: people aged 65 years and over. Volume 1: Report of the diet and nutrition survey. London, Her Majesty's Stationery Office, 1998.

[18] Yong LC, Brown CC, Schatzkin A, Dresser CM, Slesinski MJ, Cox CS, Taylor PR. Intake of vitamins E, C, and A and risk of lung cancer. *Am. J. Epidemiol.* 1997;146:231–243.

[19] Byers T, Mouchawar J. Antioxidants and cancer prevention in 1997. In: Paoletti R et al, eds. Vitamin C: the state of the art in disease prevention sixty years after the Nobel Prize. Milan, Springer. 1998. pp.29–40.

[20] Schorah CJ. Vitamin C and gastric cancer prevention. In: Paoletti R et al, eds. Vitamin C: the state of the art in disease prevention sixty years after the Nobel Prize. Milan, Springer. 1998. pp.41–49.

[21] Blot WJ, Li JY, Taylor PR, Guo W, Dawsey S, Wang GQ, Yang CS, Zheng SF, Gail M, Li GY, Yu Y, Liu B, Tangrea J, Sun Y, Liu F, Fraumeni JF, Zhang J, Li B. Nutrition intervention trials in Linxian, China: supplementation with specific vitamin/mineral combinations, cancer incidence, and disease-specific mortality in the general population. *J. Natl. Cancer Inst.* 1993;85:1483–1492.

[22] Greenberg ER, Baron JA, Tosteson TD, Freeman DH Jr, Beck GJ, Bond JH, Colacchio TA, Coller JA, Frankl HD, Haile RW, Mandel JS, Nierenberg DW, Rothstein R, Snover DC, Stevens MM, Summers RW, van Stolk RU. A clinical trial of antioxidant vitamins to prevent

colorectal adenoma. Polyp Prevention Study Group. *N. Engl. J. Med.* 1994,331:141–147.

[23] Pauling L. How to live longer and feel better. New York, *Avon Books*. 1986.

[24] Levine M, Conry-Cantilena C, Wang Y, Welch RW, Washko PW, Dhariwal KR, Park JB, Lazarev A, Graumlich JF, King J, Cantilena LR. Vitamin C pharmacokinetics in healthy volunteers: evidence for a Recommended Dietary Allowance. *Proc. Natl. Acad. Sci. U. S. A.* 1996, 93:3704–3709.

[25] Levine M, Rumsey SC, Daruwala R, Park JB, Wang Y. Criteria and recommendations for vitamin C intake. *JAMA*. 1999;281:1415-1423.

[26] Levine M, Wang Y, Padayatty SJ, Morrow J. A new recommended dietary allowance of vitamin C for healthy young women. *Proc. Natl. Acad. Sci. U. S. A.* 2001;98:9842-9846.

[27] Duconge J, Miranda-Massari JR, Gonzalez MJ, Jackson JA, Warnock W, Riordan NH. Pharmacokinetics of vitamin C: insights into the oral and intravenous administration of ascorbate. P R *Health Sci. J.* 2008;27:7-19.

[28] Nishikimi M, Yagi K. Biochemistry and molecular biology of ascorbic acid biosynthesis. *Subcell. Biochem.* 1996;25:17–39.

[29] Padayatty SJ, Katz A, Wang Y, Eck P, Kwon O, Lee JH, Chen S, Corpe C, Dutta A, Dutta SK, Levine M. Vitamin C as an antioxidant: evaluation of its role in disease prevention. *J. Am. Coll Nutr.* 2003;22:18-35.

[30] Chatterjee IB, Chatterjee GC, Ghosh NC, Ghosh JJ, Guha BC. Biological synthesis of l-ascorbic acid in animal tissues: conversion of L-gulonolactone into L-ascorbic acid. *Biochem. J.* 1960a;74:193–203.

[31] Chatterjee IB, Chatterjee GC, Ghosh NC, Ghosh JJ, Guha BC. Biological synthesis of l-ascorbic acid in animal tissues: conversion of D-glucuronolactone and L-gulonolactone into L-ascorbic acid. *Biochem. J.* 1960b;76:279–292.

[32] Nishikimi M, Fukuyama R, Minoshima S, Shimizu N, Yagi K. Cloning and chromosomal mapping of the human nonfunctional gene for L-gulonogamma-lactone oxidase, the enzyme for L-ascorbic acid biosynthesis missing in man. *J. Biol. Chem.* 1994;269:13685–13688.

[33] Nishikimi M, Kawai T, Yagi K. Guinea pigs possess a highly mutated gene for L-gulono-gammalactone oxidase, the key enzyme for L-ascorbic acid biosynthesis missing in this species. *J. Biol. Chem.* 1992;267:21967–21972.

[34] Buettner GR. The pecking order of free radicals and antioxidants: lipid peroxidation, alpha-tocopherol, and ascorbate. *Arch. Biochem. Biophys.* 1993;300:535–543.

[35] Buettner GR, Jurkiewicz BA. Ascorbate free radical as a marker of oxidative stress: an EPR study. Free Radic Biol Med. 1993;14:49–55.

[36] Buettner GR, Jurkiewicz BA. Catalytic metals, ascorbate and free radicals: combinations to avoid. *Radiat. Res*. 1996;145:532–541.

[37] Linster CL, Van Schaftingen E. Vitamin C Biosynthesis, recycling and degradation in mammals. *FEBS J.* 2007;274:1-22.

[38] Padayatty SJ, Sun H, Wang Y, Riordan HD, Hewitt SM, Katz A, Wesley RA, Levine M. Vitamin C pharmacokinetics: implications for oral and intravenous use. *Ann. Intern. Med.* 2004;140:533–537.

[39] McCormick DB, Zhang Z. Cellular assimilation of water-soluble vitamins in the mammal: riboflavin, B6, biotin and C. *Proc. Soc. Exp. Biol. Med.* 1993;202:265-270.

[40] Kallner A, Hartmann D, Horning D. Steady-state turnover and body pool of ascorbic acid in man. *Am. J. Clin. Nutr.* 1979;32:530-539.

[41] Levine GN, Frei B, Koulouris SN, Gerhard MD, Keaney JF Jr, Vita JA. Ascorbic acid reverses endothelial vasomotor dysfunction in patients with coronary artery disease. *Circulation.* 1996;93 1107–1113.

[42] Graumlich JF, Ludden TM, Conry-Cantilena C, Cantilena LR Jr, Wang Y, Levine M. Pharmacokinetic model of ascorbic acid in humans during depletion and repletion. *Pharm. Res.* 1997;14:1133-1139.

[43] Hickey DS, Roberts HJ, Cathcart RF. Dynamic Flow: A New Model for Ascorbate. *J. Orthomol. Med.* 2005;20:237-244.

[44] Wang Y, Mackenzie B, Tsukaguchi H, Weremowicz S, Morton CC, Hediger MA. Human vitamin C (L-ascorbic acid) transporter SVCT1. *Biochem. Biophys. Res. Commun.* 2000;267:488-494.

[45] Takanaga H, Mackenzue B, Hediger MA. Sodium-dependent ascorbic acid transporter family SLC23. *Pflugers Arch.* 2004;447:677-668.

[46] Hardman JG, Limbird LE, Gilman AG. Goodman, Gilman's The Pharmacological Basis of Therapeutics, 10th edition. New York, McGraw-Hill Professional. 2001.

[47] Johnston CS, Luo B. Comparison of the absorption and excretion of three commercially available sources of vitamin C. *J. Am. Diet. Assoc.* 1994;94:779-781.

[48] Mangels AR, Block G, Frey CM, Patterson BH, Taylor PR, Norkus EP, Levander OA. The bioavailability to humans of ascorbic acid from

oranges, orange juice and cooked broccoli is similar to that of synthetic ascorbic acid. *J. Nutr.* 1993;123:1054-61.

[49] Cathcart RF. Vitamin C, titrating to bowel tolerance, anascorbemia and acute induced scurvy. *Med. Hypotheses.* 1981;7:1359-1376.

[50] Mayersohn M. Vitamin C bioavailability. *J. Nutr. Sci. Vitaminol.* (Tokyo). 1992;Spec No:446-449.

[51] Kashihara T, Kitamori N, Murata A. Plasma Concentration-Time Profiles and Pharmacokinetic Analyses of Vitamin C. *Bull. Fac. Agr., Saga Univ.* 1996; 80:77-83.

[52] Bluck L, Jones K, Coward WA, Bates C. The 'anomalous' absorption of labelled and unlabelled vitamin C in man. *Br. J. Nutr.* 2005;93:627–632.

[53] Harrison FE, May JM. Vitamin C function in the brain: vital role of the ascorbate transporter SVCT2. *Free Radic. Biol. Med.* 2009;46:719-30.

[54] McColl KE. Effect of proton pump inhibitors on vitamins and iron. *Am. J. Gastroenterol.* 2009;104:2:S5-9.

[55] Banhegyi G, Braun L, Csala M, Puskas F, Mandl J. Ascorbate Metabolism and Its Regulation in Animals. *Free Radic. Biol. Med.* 1997;23:793-803.

[56] Jackson TS, Xu AM, Vita JA, Keaney JF Jr. Ascorbate prevents the interaction of superoxide and nitric oxide only at very high physiological concentrations. *Circ. Res.* 1998;83:916–922.

[57] Arrigoni O;De Tullio MC. Ascorbic acid: much more than just an antioxidant. *Biochim. Biophys. Acta Gen. Subj.* 2002;1569:1–9.

[58] May JM, Qu ZC. Transport and intracellular accumulation of vitamin C in endothelial cells: relevance to collagen synthesis. *Arch. Biochem. Biophys.* 2005;434:178–186.

[59] Tsukaguchi H, Tokui T, Mackenzie B, Berger UV, Chen XZ, Wang YX, Brubaker RF, Hediger MA. A family of mammalian Na+-dependent L-ascorbic acid transporters. *Nature.* 1999;399:70–75.

[60] Corpe C, Tu H,Wang J, Eck P,Wang Y, Schnermann J, Faulhaber-Walter R, Nussbaum R, Levine M. SVCT1 (Slc23a1) knockout mice: Slc23a1 as the vitamin C kidney reabsorptive transporter. *FASEB J.* 2008;21:LB111.

[61] Daruwala R, Song J, Koh WS, Rumsey SC, Levine M. Cloning and functional characterization of the human sodium-dependent vitamin C transporters hSVCT1 and hSVCT2. *FEBS Lett.* 1999;460: 480–484.

[62] Sotiriou S, Gispert S, Cheng J, Wang Y, Chen A, Hoogstraten-Miller S, Miller GF, Kwon O, Levine M, Guttentag SH, Nussbaum RL. Ascorbic-

acid transporter Slc23a1 is essential for vitamin C transport into the brain and for perinatal survival. *Nat. Med.* 2002;8:514–517.

[63] Castro M, Caprile T, Astuya A, Millán C, Reinicke K, Vera JC, Vásquez O, Aguayo LG, Nualart F. High-affinity sodium-vitamin C co-transporters (SVCT) expression in embryonic mouse neurons. *J. Neurochem.* 2001;78:815–823.

[64] May JM, Li L, Hayslett K, Qu ZC. Ascorbate transport and recycling by SHSY5Y neuroblastoma cells: response to glutamate toxicity. *Neurochem. Res.* 2006;31:785–794.

[65] O'Neill RD, Fillenz M, Sundstrom L, Rawlins JN. Voltammetrically monitored brain ascorbate as an index of excitatory amino acid release in the unrestrained rat. *Neurosci. Lett.* 1984;52:227–233.

[66] Rose RC, Bode AM. Biology of free radical scavengers: an evaluation of ascorbate. *FASEB J.* 1993;7:1135–1142.

[67] Grünewald RA. Ascorbic acid in the brain. *Brain Res. Rev.* 1993;18:123–133.

[68] Milby K, Oke A, Adams RN. Detailed mapping of ascorbate distribution in rat brain. *Neurosci. Lett.* 1982;28:169–174.

[69] Spector R, Lorenzo AV. Ascorbic acid homeostasis in the central nervous system. *Am. J. Physiol.* 1973;225:757–763.

[70] Godoy A, Ormazabal V, Moraga-Cid G, Zúñiga FA, Sotomayor P, Barra V, Vasquez O, Montecinos V, Mardones L, Guzmán C, Villagrán M, Aguayo LG, Oñate SA, Reyes AM, Cárcamo JG, Rivas CI, Vera JC. Mechanistic insights and functional determinants of the transport cycle of the ascorbic acid transporter SVCT2. Activation by sodium and absolute dependence on bivalent cations. *J. Biol. Chem.* 2007;282:615-24.

[71] MacDonald L, Thumser AE, Sharp P. Decreased expression of the vitamin C transporter SVCT1 by ascorbic acid in a human intestinal epithelial cell line. *Br. J. Nutr.* 2002;87: 97–100.

[72] Savini I, Rossi A, Catani MV, Ceci R, Avigliano L. Redox regulation of vitamin C transporter SVCT2 in C2C12 myotubes. *Biochem. Biophys. Res. Commun.* 2007a;361:385–390.

[73] Savini I, Catani MV, Arnone R, Rossi A, Frega G, Del Principe D, Avigliano L. Translational control of the ascorbic acid transporter SVCT2 in human platelets. *Free Radic. Biol. Med.* 2007b;42:608–616.

[74] Vera JC, Rivas CI, Fischbarg J, Golde DW. Mammalian facilitative hexose transporters mediate the transport of dehydroascorbic acid. *Nature.* 1993;364:79–82.

[75] Wilson JX. Regulation of vitamin C transport. *Annu. Rev. Nutr.* 2005;25:105–125.

[76] Angulo C, Castro MA, Rivas CI, Segretain D, Maldonado R, Yañez AJ, Slebe JC, Vera JC, Concha I. Molecular identification and functional characterization of the vitamin C transporters expressed by Sertoli cells. *J. Cell. Physiol.* 2008;217:708–716.

[77] Rumsey SC, Kwon O, Xu GW, Burant CF, Simpson I, Levine M. Glucose transporter isoforms GLUT1 and GLUT3 transport dehydroascorbic acid. *J. Biol. Chem.* 1997;272:18982–18989.

[78] DiLabio GA, Wright JS. Hemiketal formation of dehydroascorbic acid drives ascorbyl radical anion disproportionation. *Free Radic. Biol. Med.* 2000;29:480–485.

[79] Pastore P, Rizzetto T, Curcuruto O, Cin MD, Zaramella A, Marton D. Characterization of dehydroascorbic acid solutions by liquid chromatography/ mass spectrometry. *Rapid Commun. Mass Spectrom.* 2001;15:2051–2057.

[80] Deutsch JC. Dehydroascorbic acid. J. Chromatogr. A. 2000;881:299–307.

[81] Liang WJ, Johnson D, Jarvis SM. Vitamin C transport systems of mammalian cells. *Mol. Membr. Biol.* 2001;18:87–95.

[82] Reiber H, Ruff M, Uhr M. Ascorbate concentration in human cerebrospinal fluid (CSF) and serum: intrathecal accumulation and CSF flow rate. *Clin. Chim. Acta.* 1993;217:163–173.

[83] Upston JM, Karjalainen A, Bygrave FL, Stocker R. Efflux of hepatic ascorbate: a potential contributor to the maintenance of plasma vitamin C. *Biochem. J.* 1999;342:49–56.

[84] Davis KA, Samson SE, Best K, Mallhi KK, Szewczyk M, Wilson JX, Kwan CY, Grover AK. Ca(2+)-mediated ascorbate release from coronary artery endothelial cells. *Br. J. Pharmacol.* 2006;147:131–139.

[85] Rebec GV, Pierce RC. A vitamin as neuromodulator: ascorbate release into the extracellular fluid of the brain regulates dopaminergic and glutamatergic transmission. *Prog. Neurobiol.* 1994;43:537–565.

[86] Mendiratta, S, Qu, Z.-C, May JM. Erythrocyte ascorbate recycling: antioxidant effects in blood. Free Radic. Biol. Med. 1998;24:789–797.

[87] Bielski BH, Allen AO, Schwarz HA. Mechanism of disproportionation of ascorbate radicals. *J. Am. Chem. Soc.* 1981;103:3516–3518.

[88] Iyanagi T, Yamazaki I. One-electron-transfer reactions in biochemical systems. III. One-electron reduction of quinones by microsomal flavin enzymes. *Biochim. Biophys. Acta.* 1969;172:370–381.

[89] May JM, Cobb CE, Mendiratta S, Hill KE, Burk RF. Reduction of the ascorbyl free radical to ascorbate by thioredoxin reductase. *J. Biol. Chem.* 1998;273:23039–23045.

[90] Njus D, Kelley PM. The secretory-vesicle ascorbate-regenerating system: a chain of concerted H+/ e–-transfer reactions. *Biochim. Biophys. Acta.* 1993;1144:235–248.

[91] Fleming PJ, Kent UM. Cytochrome b561, ascorbic acid, and transmembrane electron transfer. *Am. J. Clin. Nutr.* 1991;54:1173S–1178S.

[92] Diliberto EJ Jr, Dean G, Carter C, Allen PL. Tissue, subcellular, and submitochondrial distributions of semidehydroascorbate reductase: possible role of semidehydroascorbate reductase in cofactor regeneration. *J. Neurochem.* 1982;39:563–568.

[93] Njus D, Kelley PM, Harnadek GJ, Pacquing YV. Mechanism of ascorbic acid regeneration mediated by cytochrome b561. *Ann. N.Y. Acad. Sci.* 1987;493:108–119.

[94] May JM, Qu ZC, Cobb CE. Extracellular reduction of the ascorbate free radical by human erythrocytes. *Biochem. Biophys. Res. Commun.* 2000;267:118–123.

[95] Van Duijn MM, Buijs JT, Van der Zee J, Van den Broek PJ. The ascorbate: ascorbate free radical oxidoreductase from the erythrocyte membrane is not cytochrome b561. *Protoplasma.* 2001;217:94–100.

[96] Winkler BS, Orselli SM, Rex TS. The redox couple between glutathione and ascorbic acid: a chemical and physiological perspective. *Free Radic. Biol. Med.* 1994;17:333–349.

[97] Wells WW, Xu DP, Yang Y, Rocque PA. Mammalian thioltransferase (glutaredoxin) and protein disulfide isomerase have dehydroascorbate reductase activity. *J. Biol. Chem.* 1990;265:15361–15364.

[98] Hellman L, Burns JJ. Metabolism of L-ascorbic acid-1-C14 in man. *J. Biol. Chem.* 1958;230:923–930.

[99] Bode AM, Cunningham L, Rose RC. Spontaneous decay of oxidized ascorbic acid (dehydrol-ascorbic acid) evaluated by high-pressure liquid chromatography. *Clin. Chem.* 1990;36:1807–1809.

[100] Simpson GL, Ortwerth BJ. The non-oxidative degradation of ascorbic acid at physiological conditions. *Biochim. Biophys. Acta.* 2000;1501:12–24.

[101] Tolbert BM, Ward JB. Dehydroascorbic acid, in: Seib P.A, Tolbert B.M. (Eds), Ascorbic acid: chemistry, metabolism, and uses. Washington, DC, American Chemical Society. 1982. pp. 101–123.

[102] Koshiishi I, Mamura Y, Liu J, Imanari T. Degradation of dehydroascorbate to 2,3-diketogulonate in blood circulation. *Biochim. Biophys. Acta.* 1998;1425:209–214.

[103] Rodrigo R, Guichard C, Charles R. Clinical pharmacology and therapeutic use of antioxidant vitamins. *Fundam. Clin. Pharmacol.* 2007;21:111–127.

[104] Dizdaroglu M, Jaruga P, Birincioglu M, Rodriguez H. Free radical-induced damage to DNA: mechanisms and measurement. *Free Radic. Biol. Med.* 2002;32 1102–1115.

[105] Milne GL, Musiek ES, Morrow JD. F2-isoprostanes as markers of oxidative stress in vivo: an overview. *Biomarkers.* 2005;10:S10–S23.

[106] Reznick AZ, Packer L. Oxidative damage to proteins: spectrophotometric method for carbonyl assay. *Methods Enzymol.* 1994;233:357–363.

[107] Galley HF, Davies MJ, Webster NR. Ascorbyl radical formation in patients with sepsis: effect of ascorbate loading. *Free Radic. Biol. Med.* 1996;20:139–143.

[108] Niki E, Noguchi N, Tsuchihashi H, Gotoh N. Interaction among vitamin C, vitamin E, and β-carotene. *Am. J. Clin. Nutr.* 1995;62:1322S–1326S.

[109] May JM, Qu ZC, Mendiratta S. Protection and recycling of α-tocopherol in human erythrocytes by intracellular ascorbic acid. *Arch. Biochem. Biophys.* 1998;349:281–289.

[110] Carr AC, Zhu BZ, Frei B. Potential antiatherogenic mechanisms of ascorbate (vitamin C) and alpha-tocopherol (vitamin E). *Circ. Res.* 2000;87:349-354.

[111] Kovachich GB, Mishra OP. The effect of ascorbic acid on malonaldehyde formation, K+, Na+ andwater content of brain slices. *Exp. Brain Res.* 1983;50:62–68.

[112] Bano S, Parihar MS. Reduction of lipid peroxidation in different brain regions by a combination of α-tocopherol and ascorbic acid. *J. Neural Transm.* 1997;104:1277–1286.

[113] Aguirre R, May M. Inflammation in the Vascular Bed: Importance of Vitamin C. *Pharmacol Ther.* 2008;119:96–103.

[114] Rodrigo R. Oxidative Stress and Antioxidants, 1st edition. New York, Nova Publishers. 2009a.

[115] Prockop DJ, Kivirikko KI. Collagens: molecular biology, diseases, and potentials for therapy. *Annu. Rev. Biochem.* 1995;64:403–434.

[116] Rebouche CJ. Ascorbic acid and carnitine biosynthesis. *Am. J. Clin. Nutr.* 1991;54:S1147–S1152.

[117] Levine RL, Stadtman ER. Oxidative modification of proteins during aging. *Exp. Gerontol.* 2001;36:1495–1502.

[118] Eipper BA, Milgram SL, Husten EJ, Yun HY, Mains RE. Peptidylglycine alpha amidating monooxygenase: a multifunctional protein with catalytic, processing, and routing domains. *Protein Sci.* 1993;2:489-497.

[119] Eipper BA, Stoffers DA, Mains RE. The biosynthesis of neuropeptides: peptide alpha amidation. *Annu. Rev. Neurosci.* 1992;15:57–85.

[120] Englard S, Seifter S. The biochemical functions of ascorbic acid. *Annu. Rev. Nutr.* 1986;6:365–406.

[121] Bornstein SR, Yoshida-Hiroi M, Sotiriou S, Levine M, Hartwig HG, Nussbaum RL, Eisenhofer G. Impaired adrenal catecholamine system function in mice with deficiency of the ascorbic acid transporter (SVCT2). *FASEB J.* 2003;17:1928-1930.

[122] Njus D, Knoth J, Cook C, Kelley PM. Electron transfer across the chromaffin granule membrane. *J. Biol. Chem.* 1983;258:27–30.

[123] Wakefield LM, Cass AE, Radda GK. Electron transfer across the chromaffin granule membrane: use of EPR to demonstrate reduction of intravesicular ascorbate radical by the extravesicular mitochondrial NADH:ascorbate radical oxidoreductase. *J. Biol. Chem.* 1986;261:9746–9752.

[124] Levine M, Asher A, Pollard H, Zinder O. Ascorbic acid and catecholamine secretion from cultured chromaffin cells. *J. Biol. Chem.* 1983;258:13111–13115.

[125] Padayatty SJ, Doppman JL, Chang R, Wang Y, Gill J, Papanicolaou DA, Levine M. Human adrenal glands secrete vitamin C in response to adrenocorticotrophic hormone. *Am. J. Clin. Nutr.* 2007;86:145–149.

[126] Sandstrom MI, Rebec GV. Extracellular ascorbate modulates glutamate dynamics: role of behavioral activation. *BMC Neurosci.* 2007;8:32.

[127] Kiyatkin EA, Rebec GV. Ascorbate modulates glutamate-induced excitations of striatal neurons. *Brain Res.* 1998;812:14–22.

[128] Rebec GV, Witowski SR, Sandstrom MI, Rostand RD, Kennedy RT. Extracellular ascorbate modulates cortically evoked glutamate dynamics in rat striatum. *Neurosci. Lett.* 2005;378:166–170.

[129] Ciani E, Groneng L, Voltattorni M, Rolseth V, Contestabile A, Paulsen RE. Inhibition of free radical production or free radical scavenging protects from the excitotoxic cell death mediated by glutamate in cultures of cerebellar granule neurons. *Brain Res.* 1996;728:1–6.

[130] Atlante A, Gagliardi S, Minervini GM, Ciotti MT, Marra E, Calissano P. Glutamate neurotoxicity in rat cerebellar granule cells: a major role for xanthine oxidase in oxygen radical formation. *J. Neurochem.* 1997;68:2038–2045.

[131] Majewska MD, Bell JA, London ED. Regulation of the NMDA receptor by redox phenomena: inhibitory role of ascorbate. *Brain Res.* 1990;537:328–332.

[132] Hillered L, Persson L, Bolander HG, Hallstrom A, Ungerstedt U. Increased extracellular levels of ascorbate in the striatum after middle cerebral artery occlusion in the rat monitored by intracerebral microdialysis. *Neurosci. Lett.* 1988;95:286–290.

[133] Rice ME. Ascorbate regulation and its neuroprotective role in the brain. *Trends Neurosci.* 2000;23:209–216.

[134] Yusa T. Increased extracellular ascorbate release reflects glutamate re-uptake during the early stage of reperfusion after forebrain ischemia in rats. *Brain Res.* 2001;897:104–113.

[135] Kuo CH, Hata F, Yoshida H, Yamatodani A, Wada H. Effect of ascorbic acid on release of acetylcholine from synaptic vesicles prepared from different species of animals and release of noradrenaline from synaptic vesicles of rat brain. *Life Sci.* 1979;24:911–915.

[136] Dhingra D, Parle M, Kulkarni SK. Comparative brain cholinesterase-inhibiting activity of Glycyrrhiza glabra, Myristica fragrans, ascorbic acid, and metrifonate in mice. *J. Med. Food.* 2006;9:281–283.

[137] Miller BT, Cicero TJ. Ascorbic acid enhances the release of luteinizing hormone-releasing hormone from the mediobasal hypothalamus in vitro. *Life Sci.* 1986;39:2447–2454.

[138] Eldridge CF, Bunge MB, Bunge RP, Wood PM. Differentiation of axon-related Schwann cells in vitro. I. Ascorbic acid regulates basal lamina assembly and myelin formation. *J. Cell Biol.* 1987;105:1023–1034.

[139] Ulker S, McKeown PP, Bayraktutan U. Vitamins reverse endothelial dysfunction through regulation of eNOS and NAD(P)H oxidase activities. *Hypertension.* 2003;41:534-539.

[140] Böhm F, Settergren M, Pernow J. Vitamin C blocks vascular dysfunction and release of interleukin-6 induced by endothelin-1 in humans in vivo. *Atherosclerosis.* 2007;190:408-415.

[141] Jialal I, Grundy SM. Preservation of the endogenous antioxidants in low density lipoprotein by ascorbate but not probucol during oxidative modification. *J. Clin. Invest.* 1991;87:597–601.

[142] Semenza GL. HIF-1, O(2), and the 3 PHDs: how animal cells signal hypoxia to the nucleus. *Cell.* 2001;107:1–3.
[143] Schorah CJ, Sobala GM, Sanderson M, Collis N, Primrose JN. Gastric juice ascorbic acid: effects of disease and implications for gastric carcinogenesis. *Am. J. Clin. Nutr.* 1991;53:287S-293S.
[144] Correa P. Human gastric carcinogenesis: a multistep and multifactorial process. First American Cancer Society Award Lecture on Cancer Epidemiology and Prevention. *Cancer Res.* 1992;52:6735–6740.
[145] Byers T, Guerrero N. Epidemiologic evidence for vitamin C and vitamin E in cancer prevention. *Am. J. Clin. Nutr.* 1995;62:S1385–S1392.
[146] Hallberg L, Brune M, Rossander-Hulthen L. Is there a physiological role of vitamin C in iron absorption? *Ann. N. Y. Acad. Sci.* 1987;498:324–332.
[147] Hallberg L. Wheat fiber, phytates and iron absorption. *Scand. J. Gastroenterol.* 1987;129:S73–S79.
[148] Stokes PL, Melikian V, Leeming RL, Portman-Graham H, Blair JA, Cooke WT. Folate metabolism in scurvy. *Am. J. Clin. Nutr.* 1975;28:126-129.
[149] McLaren DS. A colour atlas of nutritional disorders. London, Wolfe Medical Publications. 1992.
[150] Bartley W, Krebs HA, O'Brien JRP. Vitamin C requirements of human adults. London, Her Majesty's Stationery Office. 1953. *Medical Research Council Special Report Series No.* 280.
[151] Krebs NA, Peters RA, Coward KH. Vitamin C requirement of human adults: experimental study of vitamin C deprivation in man. *Lancet,* 1948, 254:853–858.
[152] Baker EM, Hodges RE, Hood J, Sauberlich HE, March SC. Metabolism of ascorbic-1–14C acid in experimental human scurvy. *Am. J. Clin. Nutr.* 1969;22:549-558.
[153] Baker EM, Hodges RE, Hood J, Sauberlich HE, March SC, Canham JE. Metabolism of 14C- and 3H-labeled L-ascorbic acid in human scurvy. *Am. J. Clin. Nutr.* 1971;24:444-454.
[154] Lee W, Davis KA, Rettmer RL, Labbe RF. Ascorbic acid status: biochemical and clinical considerations. *Am. J. Clin. Nutr.* 1988;48:286-90.
[155] Cameron E, Pauling L. Cancer and Vitamin C. Philadelphia, *Camino Books.* 1993.
[156] Canoy D, Wareham N, Welch A, Bingham S, Luben R, Day N, Khaw K. Plasma ascorbic acid concentrations and fat distribution in 19,068

British men and women in the European Prospective Investigation into Cancer and Nutrition Norfolk cohort study. *Am. J. Clin. Nutr.* 2005;82:1203–1209.

[157] Bsoul S, Terezhalmy G. Vitamin C in health and disease. *J. Contemp. Dent. Pract.* 2004;5:1-13.

[158] Lassègue B, Griendling KK. Reactive oxygen species in hypertension. *Am. J. Hypertens.* 2004;17:852–860.

[159] Rodrigo R, Passalacqua W, Araya J, Orellana M, Rivera G. Implications of oxidative stress and homocysteine in the pathophysiology of essential hypertension. *J. Cardiovasc. Pharmacol.* 2003;42:453–461.

[160] Bengtsson SH, Gulluyan LM, Dusting GJ, Drummond GR. Novel isoforms of NADPH oxidase in vascular physiology and pathophysiology. *Clin. Exp. Pharmacol. Physiol.* 2003;30:849–854.

[161] Redon J, Oliva MR, Tormos C, Giner V, Chaves J, Iradi A, Saez GT. Antioxidant activities and oxidative stress byproducts in human hypertension. *Hypertension.* 2003;41:1096–1101.

[162] Houston MC. Nutraceuticals, vitamins, antioxidants, and minerals in the prevention and treatment of hypertension. *Prog. Cardiovasc. Dis.* 2005;47:396–449.

[163] Lacy F, Kailasam M.T, O'Connor D.T, Schmid-Schonbein G.W, Parmer R.J. Plasma hydrogen peroxide production in human essential hypertension: role of heredity, gender, and ethnicity. *Hypertension.* 2000;36 878–884.

[164] Stojiljkovic MP, Lopes HF, Zhang D, Morrow JD, Goodfriend TL, Egan BM. Increasing plasma fatty acids elevates F2-isoprostanes in humans: implications for the cardiovascular risk factor cluster. *J. Hypertens.* 2002;201:1215–1221.

[165] Kashyap MK, Yadav V, Sherawat BS, Jain S, Kumari S, Khullar M, Sharma PC, Nath R. Different antioxidants status, total antioxidant power and free radicals in essential hypertension. *Mol. Cell. Biochem.* 2005;277:89–99.

[166] Wattanapitayakul SK, Bauer JA. Oxidative pathways in cardiovascular disease: roles, mechanisms, and therapeutic implications. *Pharmacol. Ther.* 2001;89:187–206.

[167] John S, Schmieder RE. Potential mechanisms of impaired endothelial function in arterial hypertension and hypercholesterolemia. *Curr. Hypertens. Rep.* 2003;5:199–207.

[168] Dusting GJ, Fennessy P, Yin ZL, Gurevich V. Nitric oxide in atherosclerosis: vascular protector or villain? *Clin. Exp. Pharmacol.* Physiol. 1998;25:S34–S41.

[169] Dusting GJ, Dart A. Endothelial dysfunction associated with cardiovascular disease and transplantation. In: Griffith D.T, Mathie R., Eds.. The haemodynamic effects of nitric oxide. London, World Scientific Publishing. 1999. pp. 410–433.

[170] Zicha J, Dobesova Z, Kunes J. Relative deficiency of nitric oxide-dependent vasodilation in salt- hypertensive Dahl rats: the possible role of superoxide anions. *J. Hypertens.* 2001;19:247–254.

[171] Babior B.M. Nadph oxidase: an update. *Blood.* 1999;93:1464–1476.

[172] Ray R, Shah AM. Nadph oxidase and endothelial cell function. *Clin. Sci.* (Lond.) 2005;109:217–226.

[173] Wilcox CS. Oxidative stress and nitric oxide deficiency in the kidney: a critical link to hypertension? *Am. J. Physiol. Regul. Integr. Comp. Physiol.* 2005;289:R913–R935.

[174] Ellmark SH, Dusting GJ, Fui MN, Guzzo-Pernell N, Drummond GR. The contribution of Nox4 to NADPH oxidase activity in mouse vascular smooth muscle. *Cardiovasc. Res.* 2005;65:495–504.

[175] Zhan CD, Sindhu RK, Pang J, Ehdaie A, Vaziri ND. Superoxide dismutase, catalase and glutathione peroxidase in the spontaneously hypertensive rat kidney: effect of antioxidant-rich diet. *J. Hypertens.* 2004;22:2025–2033.

[176] Yokoyama T, Date C, Kokubo Y, Yoshiike N, Matsumura Y, Tanaka H. Serum vitamin C concentration was inversely associated with subsequent 20-year incidence of stroke in a Japanese rural community. The Shibata study. *Stroke.* 2000;31:2287–2294.

[177] Sakai N, Yokoyama T, Date C, Yoshiike N, Matsumura Y. An inverse relationship between serum vitamin C and blood pressure in a Japanese community. *J. Nutr. Sci. Vitaminol.* (Tokyo) 1998;44:853–867.

[178] Appel LJ, Moore TJ, Obarzanek E, Vollmer WM, Svetkey LP, Sacks FM, Bray GA, Vogt TM, Cutler JA, Windhauser MM, Lin PH, Karanja N. A clinical trial of the effects of dietary patterns on blood pressure. DASH Collaborative Research Group. *N. Engl. J. Med.* 1997;336:1117–1124.

[179] Conlin PR, Chow D, Miller ER 3rd, Svetkey LP, Lin PH, Harsha DW, Moore TJ, Sacks FM, Appel LJ. The effect of dietary patterns on blood pressure control in hypertensive patients: results from the Dietary

Approaches to Stop Hypertension (DASH) trial. *Am. J. Hypertens.* 2000;13:949–955.

[180] John JH, Ziebland S, Yudkin P, Roe LS, Neil HA, Oxford Fruit and Vegetable Study Group. Effects of fruit and vegetable consumption on plasma antioxidant concentrations and blood pressure: a randomised controlled trial. *Lancet.* 2002;359:1969–1974.

[181] Nishikawa Y, Tatsumi K, Matsuura T, Yamamoto A, Nadamoto T, Urabe K. Effects of vitamin C on high blood pressure induced by salt in spontaneously hypertensive rats. *J. Nutr. Sci. Vitaminol.* (Tokyo) 2003;49:301–309.

[182] Reckelhoff JF, Kanji V, Racusen LC, Schmidt AM, Yan SD, Marrow J, Roberts LJ 2nd, Salahudeen AK. Vitamin E ameliorates enhanced renal lipid peroxidation and accumulation of F2-isoprostanes in aging kidneys. *Am. J. Physiol.* 1998;274:R767–R774.

[183] Chen X, Touyz RM, Park JB, Schiffrin EL. Antioxidant effects of vitamins C and E are associated with altered activation of vascular NADPH oxidase and superoxide dismutase in stroke- prone SHR. *Hypertension.* 2001;38:606–611.

[184] Atarashi K, Ishiyama A, Takagi M, Minami M, Kimura K, Goto A, Omata M. Vitamin E ameliorates the renal injury of Dahl Salt-sensitive rats. *Am. J. Hypertens.* 1997;10:116s–119s.

[185] Motoyama T, Kawano H, Kugiyama K, Hirashima O, Ohgushi M, Yoshimura M, Ogawa H, Yasue H. Endothelium-dependent vasodilation in the brachial artery is impaired in smokers: effect of vitamin C. *Am. J. Physiol.* 1997;273:1644–1650.

[186] Beckman JA, Goldfine AB, Gordon MB, Creager MA. Ascorbate restores endothelium-dependent vasodilation impaired by acute hyperglycemia in humans. *Circulation.* 2001;103:1618–1623.

[187] Pleiner J, Schaller G, Mittermayer F, Bayerle-Eder M, Roden M, Wolzt M. FFA-induced endothelial dysfunction can be corrected by vitamin C. *J. Clin. Endocrinol. Metab.* 2002a;87:2913-2917.

[188] Pleiner J, Mittermayer F, Schaller G, MacAllister RJ, Wolzt M. High doses of vitamin C reverse Escherichia coli endotoxin-induced hyporeactivity to acetylcholine in the human forearm. *Circulation.* 2002b;106:1460-1464.

[189] Pleiner J, Schaller G, Mittermayer F, Marsik C, MacAllister RJ, Kapiotis S, Ziegler S, Ferlitsch A, Wolzt M. Intra-arterial vitamin C prevents endothelial dysfunction caused by ischemia-reperfusion. *Atherosclerosis.* 2008;197:383-391.

[190] Schneider MP, Delles C, Schmidt BM, Oehmer S, Schwarz TK, Schmieder RE, John S. Superoxide scavenging effects of N-acetylcysteine and vitamin C in subjects with essential hypertension. *Am. J. Hypertens.* 2005;18:1111-1117.

[191] Vita JA, Frei B, Holbrook M, Gokce N, Leaf C, Keaney JF Jr. L-2-Oxothiazolidine-4-carboxylic acid reverses endothelial dysfunction in patients with coronary artery disease. *J. Clin. Invest.* 1998;101:1408–1414.

[192] Duffy SJ, Gokce N, Holbrook M, Hunter LM, Biegelsen ES, Huang A, Keaney JF Jr, Vita JA. Effect of ascorbic acid treatment on conduit vessel endothelial dysfunction in patients with hypertension. *Am. J. Physiol. Heart Circ. Physiol.* 2001;280:H528–H534.

[193] Attia DM, Verhagen AM, Stroes ES, van Faassen EE, Gröne HJ, De Kimpe SJ, Koomans HA, Braam B, Joles JA. Vitamin E alleviates renal injury, but not hypertension, during chronic nitric oxide synthase inhibition in rats. *J. Am. Soc. Nephrol.* 2001;12:2585–2593.

[194] Vásquez-Vivar J, Kalyanaraman B, Martásek P, Hogg N, Masters BS, Karoui H, Tordo P, Pritchard KA Jr. Superoxide generation by endothelial nitric oxide synthase: the influence of cofactors. *Proc. Natl. Acad. Sci. U. S. A.* 1998;95:9220–9225.

[195] Forstermann U. Endothelial NO synthase as a source of NO and superoxide. *Eur. J. Clin. Pharmacol.* 2006;62:5–12.

[196] Heller R, Werner-Felmayer G, Werner E.R. Antioxidants and endothelial nitric oxide synthesis. *Eur. J. Clin. Pharmacol.* 2006;62:21–28.

[197] Heller R, Werner-Felmayer G, Werner E.R. Alpha-tocopherol and endothelial nitric oxide synthesis. *Ann. N. Y. Acad. Sci.* 2004;1031:74–85.

[198] Czernichow S, Bertrais S, Blacher J, Galan P, Briançon S, Favier A, Safar M, Hercberg S. Effect of supplementation with antioxidants upon long-term risk of hypertension in the SU.VI.MAX study: association with plasma antioxidant levels. *J. Hypertens.* 2005;23:2013-2018.

[199] Bates CJ, Walmsley CM, Prentice A, Finch S. Does vitamin C reduce blood pressure? Results of a large study of people aged 65 or older. *J. Hypertens.* 1998;16:925–932.

[200] Fotherby MD, Williams JC, Forster LA, Craner P, Ferns GA. Effect of vitamin C on ambulatory blood pressure and plasma lipids in older persons. *J. Hypertens.* 2000;18:411–415.

[201] Block G, Mangels AR, Norkus EP, Patterson BH, Levander OA, Taylor PR. Ascorbic acid status and subsequent diastolic and systolic blood pressure. *Hypertension.* 2001;37:261–267.

[202] Ghosh SK, Ekpo EB, Shah IU, Girling AJ, Jenkins C, Sinclair AJ. A double-blind, placebo-controlled parallel trial of vitamin C treatment in elderly patients with hypertension. *Gerontology.* 1994;40:268–272.

[203] Rodrigo R. Hypertension. In: Rodrigo R, editor. Oxidative Stress and Antioxidants: Their role in Human Disease. New York, Nova Publishers. 2009b. pp. 25-62.

[204] Pryor WA, Squadrito GL. The chemistry of peroxynitrite: a product from the reaction of nitric oxide with superoxide. *Am. J. Physiol.* 1995;268:L699–L722.

[205] Willis GC. An experimental study of the intimal ground substance in atherosclerosis. *Can. Med. Assoc. J.* 1953;69:17–22.

[206] Willis GC. The reversibility of atherosclerosis. *Can. Med. Assoc. J.* 1957;77:106–108.

[207] Price KD, Price CS, Reynolds RD. Hyperglycemia-induced latent scurvy and atherosclerosis: the scorbutic-metaplasia hypothesis. *Med. Hypotheses.* 1996;46:119–129.

[208] Chevion M, Berenshtein E, Stadtman ER. Human studies related to protein oxidation: protein carbonyl content as a marker of damage. *Free Radic. Res.* 2000;33:S99–S108.

[209] Tahara S, Matsuo M, Kaneko T. Age-related changes in oxidative damage to lipids and DNA in rat skin. *Mech. Ageing Dev.* 2001;122:415–426.

[210] Stocker R, Keaney JF. Role of oxidative modifications in atherosclerosis. *Physiol. Rev.* 2004;84:1381–1478.

[211] Molina V, Rodrigo R. Atheroesclerosis. In: Rodrigo R, editor. Oxidative Stress and Antioxidants: Their role in Human Disease. New York, Nova Publishers. 2009. pp. 63-90.

[212] Deem TL, Cook-Mills JM. Vascular cell adhesion molecule 1 (VCAM-1) activation of endothelial cell matrix metalloproteinases: role of reactive oxygen species. *Blood.* 2004;104:2385–2393.

[213] Rajagopalan S, Meng XP, Ramasamy S, Harrison DG, Galis ZS. Reactive oxygen species produced by macrophage derived foam cells regulate the activity of vascular matrix metalloproteinases in vitro: implications for atherosclerotic plaque stability. *J. Clin. Invest.* 1996;98:2572–2579.

[214] Shinozaki K, Kashiwagi A, Nishio Y, Okamura T, Yoshida Y, Masada M, Toda N, Kikkawa R. Abnormal biopterin metabolism is a major cause of impaired endothelium-dependent relaxation through nitric oxide/O2) imbalance in insulin-resistant rat aorta. *Diabetes.* 1999;48:2437–2445.

[215] Salonen RM, Nyyssönen K, Kaikkonen J, Porkkala-Sarataho E, Voutilainen S, Rissanen TH, Tuomainen TP, Valkonen VP, Ristonmaa U, Lakka HM, Vanharanta M, Salonen JT, Poulsen HE. Six-year effect of combined vitamin C and E supplementation on atherosclerotic progression: the Antioxidant Supplementation in Atherosclerosis Prevention (ASAP) Study. *Circulation.* 2003;107:947–953.

[216] Dimmeler S, Hermann C, Zeiher AM. Apoptosis of endothelial cells. Contribution to the pathophysiology of atherosclerosis? *Eur.Cytokine Netw.* 1998;9:697–698.

[217] Rossig L, Dimmeler S, Zeiher AM. Apoptosis in the vascular wall and atherosclerosis. *Basic. Res.Cardiol.* 2001;96:11–22.

[218] Ho FM, Liu SH, Liau CS, Huang PJ, Lin-Shiau SY. High glucose-induced apoptosis in human endothelial cells is mediated by sequential activations of c-Jun NH2-terminal kinase and caspase-3. *Circulation.* 2000;101:2618–2624.

[219] Recchioni R, Marcheselli F, Moroni F, Pieri C. Apoptosis in human aortic endothelial cells induced by hyperglycemic condition involves mitochondrial depolarization and is prevented by N-acetyl-L-cysteine. *Metabolism.* 2002;51:1384–1388.

[220] Saeed RW, Peng T, Metz CN. Ascorbic acid blocks the growth inhibitory effect of tumor necrosis factor alpha on endothelial cells. *Exp. Biol. Med.*(Maywood.) 2003;228:855–865.

[221] Rössig L, Hoffmann J, Hugel B, Mallat Z, Haase A, Freyssinet JM, Tedgui A, Aicher A, Zeiher AM, Dimmeler S. Vitamin C inhibits endothelial cell apoptosis in congestive heart failure. *Circulation.* 2001;104:2182–2187.

[222] Yoshikawa K, Takahashi S, Imamura Y, Sado Y, Hayashi T. Secretion of non-helical collagenous polypeptides of alpha1(IV) and alpha2(IV) chains upon depletion of ascorbate by cultured human cells. *J. Biochem.* 2001;129:929–936.

[223] Libby P, Aikawa M. Vitamin C, collagen, and cracks in the plaque. *Circulation.* 2002;105:1396–1398.

[224] Aikawa M, Rabkin E, Okada Y, Voglic SJ, Clinton SK, Brinckerhoff CE, Sukhova GK, Libby P. Lipid lowering by diet reduces matrix

metalloproteinase activity and increases collagen content of rabbit atheroma: a potential mechanism of lesion stabilization. *Circulation.* 1998;97:2433–2444.

[225] Fukumoto Y, Libby P, Rabkin E, Hill CC, Enomoto M, Hirouchi Y, Shiomi M, Aikawa M. Statins alter smooth muscle cell accumulation and collagen content in established atheroma of Watanabe heritable hyperlipidemic rabbits. *Circulation.* 2001;103:993–999.

[226] Weber C, Erl W, Weber K, Weber PC. Increased adhesiveness of isolated monocytes to endothelium is prevented by vitamin C intake in smokers. *Circulation.* 1996;93:1488-1492.

[227] Adams MR, Jessup W, Celermajer DS. Cigarette smoking is associated with increased human monocyte adhesion to endothelial cells: reversibility with oral L-arginine but not vitamin C. *J. Am. Coll. Cardiol.* 1997;29:491-497.

[228] Das S, Ray R, Snehlata, Das N, Srivastava LM. Effect of ascorbic acid on prevention of hypercholesterolemia induced atherosclerosis. *Mol. Cell Biochem.* 2006;285:143-147.

[229] Fang JC, Kinlay S, Beltrame J, Hikiti H, Wainstein M, Behrendt D, Suh J, Frei B, Mudge GH, Selwyn AP, Ganz P. Effect of vitamins C and on progression of transplant-associated arteriosclerosis: a randomised trial. *Lancet.* 2002;359:1108–1113.

[230] Behrendt D, Beltrame J, Hikiti H, Wainstein M, Kinlay S, Selwyn AP, Ganz P, Fang JC. Impact of coronary endothelial function on the progression of cardiac transplant associated arteriosclerosis: effect of anti-oxidant vitamins C and E. *J. Heart Lung Transplant.* 2006;25:426–433.

[231] Ehnholm C, Tenkanen H, de Knijff P, Havekes L, Rosseneu M, Menzel HJ, Tiret L. Genetic polymorphism of apolipoprotein A-IV in five different regions of Europe. Relations to plasma lipoproteins and to history of myocardial infarction: the EARS study. European Atherosclerosis Research Study. *Atherosclerosis.* 1994;107:229–238.

[232] Morris BJ, Glenn CL, Wilcken DE, Wang XL. Influence of an inducible nitric oxide synthase promoter variant on clinical variables in patients with coronary artery disease. *Clin. Sci.* (Lond.) 2001;100:551–556.

[233] Tang Y, Taylor KT, Sobieski DA, Medved ES, Lipsky RH. Identification of a human CD36 isoform produced by exon skipping. Conservation of exon organization and pre-mRNA splicing patterns with a CD36 gene family member, CLA-1. *J. Biol. Chem.* 1994;269:6011–6015.

[234] Kern P, Kolowos W, Hagenhofer M, Frank C, Kalden J.R, Herrmann M. Alternatively spliced mRNA molecules of the thrombospondin receptor (CD36) in human PBMC. *Eur. J. Immunogenet.* 1999;26:337–342.

[235] Mohindra A, Kabi BC, Kaul N, Trivedi SS. Vitamin E and carotene status in pre-eclamptic pregnant women from India. *Panminerva Med.* 2002;44:261-264.

[236] Palan PR, Mikhail MS, Romney SL. Placental and serum levels of carotenoids in preeclampsia. *Obstet. Gynecol.* 2001;98:459-462.

[237] Palan PR, Shaban DW, Martino T, Mikhail MS. Lipid-soluble antioxidants and pregnancy: maternal serum levels of coenzyme Q10, alpha-tocopherol and gamma-tocopherol in preeclampsia and normal pregnancy. *Gynecol. Obstet. Invest.* 2004;58:8-13.

[238] Williams MA, Woelk GB, King IB, Jenkins L, Mahomed K. Plasma carotenoids, retinol, tocopherols, and lipoproteins in preeclamptic and normotensive pregnant Zimbabwean women. *Am. J. Hypertens.* 2003;16:665-672.

[239] Sankaralingam S, Arenas IA, Lalu MM, Davidge ST. Preeclampsia: current understanding of the molecular basis of vascular dysfunction. *Expert Rev. Mol. Med.* 2006;8:1–20.

[240] Rodrigo R, Parra M, Bosco C, Fernández V, Barja P, Guajardo J, Messina R. Pathophysiological basis for the prophylaxis of preeclampsia through early supplementation with antioxidant vitamins. *Pharmacol. Ther.* 2005;107:177–197.

[241] Parra M. Pre-Eclampsia. In: Rodrigo R, editor. Oxidative Stress and Antioxidants: Their role in Human Disease. New York, Nova Publishers. 2009. pp. 135-157.

[242] Nunes GL, Robinson K, Kalynych A, King SB. III, Sgoutas DS, Berk BC. Vitamins C and E inhibit O2-production in the pig coronary artery. *Circulation.* 1997;96:3593–3601.

[243] Chaudiere J, Ferrari-Iliou R. Intracellular antioxidants: from chemical to biochemical mechanisms. *Food Chem. Toxicol.* 1999;37:949–962.

[244] Taddei S, Virdis A, Ghaidoni L. Vitamin C improves endothelium-dependent vasodilation by restoring nitric oxide activity in essential hypertension. *Circulation.* 1998;97:2222–2229.

[245] Newaz MA, Nawal NN, Rohaizan CH, Muslim N, Gapor A. Alpha-tocopherol increased nitric oxide synthase activity in blood vessels of spontaneously hypertensive rats. *Am. J. Hypertens.* 1999;12:839–844.

[246] Moran JP, Cohen L, Greene JM, Xu G, Feldman EB, Hames CG, Feldman DS. Plasma ascorbic acid concentrations relate inversely to blood pressure in human subjects. *Am. J. Clin. Nutr.* 1993;57:213–217.

[247] Chappell LC, Seed PT, Briley AL, Kelly FJ, Lee R, Hunt BJ, Parmar K, Bewley SJ, Shennan AH, Steer PJ, Poston L. Effect of antioxidants on the occurrence of pre-eclampsia in women at increased risk: a randomised trial. *Lancet.* 1999;354:810–816.

[248] Beazley D, Ahokas R, Livingston J, Griggs M, Sibai BM. Vitamin C and E supplementation in women at high risk for preeclampsia: a double-blind, placebo-controlled trial. *Am. J. Obstet. Gynecol.* 2005;192:520–521.

[249] Rumbold AR, Crowther CA, Haslam RR, Dekker GA, Robinson JS, ACTS Study Group. Vitamins C and E and the risks of preeclampsia and perinatal complications. *N. Engl. J. Med.* 2006;354:1796–1806.

[250] Poston L, Briley AL, Seed PT, Kelly FJ, Shennan AH. Vitamins in Pre-eclampsia (VIP) Trial Consortium. Vitamin C and vitamin E in pregnant women at risk for pre-eclampsia (VIP trial): randomised placebo-controlled trial. *Lancet.* 2006;367:1145–1154.

[251] Vita JA, Keaney JF Jr, Raby KE, Morrow JD, Freedman JE, Lynch S, Koulouris SN, Hankin BR, Frei B. Low plasma ascorbic acid independently predicts the presence of an unstable coronary syndrome. *J. Am. Coll. Cardiol.* 1998;31:980–986.

[252] Roberts JM, Lain KY. Recent Insights into the pathogenesis of pre-eclampsia. *Placenta.* 2002;23:359–372.

[253] Librach CL, Werb Z, Fitzgerald ML, Chiu K, Corwin NM, Esteves RA, Grobelny D, Galardy R, Damsky CH, Fisher SJ. 92-kD type IV collagenase mediates invasion of human cytotrophoblasts. *J. Cell. Biol.* 1991;113:437–449.

[254] Braekke K, Holthe MR, Harsem NK, Fagerhol MK, Staff AC. Calprotectin, a marker of inflammation, is elevated in the maternal but not in the fetal circulation in preeclampsia. *Am. J. Obstet. Gynecol.* 2005;193:227–233.

[255] Zhou Y, Damsky CH, Fisher SJ.Preeclampsia is associated with failure of human cytotrophoblasts to mimic a vascular adhesion phenotype. One cause of defective endovascular invasion in this syndrome? *J. Clin. Invest.* 1997;99:2152–2164.

[256] Cui XL, Brockman D, Campos B, Myatt L. Expression of NADPH oxidase isoform 1 (Nox1) in human placenta: involvement in preeclampsia. *Placenta.* 2006;27:422–431.

[257] Fiore G, Florio P, Micheli L, Nencini C, Rossi M, Cerretani D, Ambrosini G, Giorgi G, Petraglia F. Endothelin-1 triggers placental oxidative stress pathways: putative role in preeclampsia. *J. Clin. Endocrinol. Metab.* 2005;90:4205–4210.

[258] Lindheimer M.D, Sibai B.M. Antioxidant supplementation in pre-eclampsia. *Lancet.* 2006;367:1119–1120.

[259] Bodnar LM, Tang G, Ness RB, Harger G, Roberts JM. Periconceptional multivitamin use reduces the risk of preeclampsia. *Am. J. Epidemiol.* 2006;164:470–477.

[260] Rodrigo R, Vinay J, Castillo R, Cereceda M, Asenjo R, Zamorano J, Araya J, Castillo-Koch R, Espinoza J, Larraín E. Use of vitamins C and E as a prophylactic therapy to prevent postoperative atrial fibrillation. *Int. J. Cardiol.* 2010;138:221-228.

[261] Carnes CA, Chung MK, Nakayama T, Nakayama H, Baliga RS, Piao S, Kanderian A, Pavia S, Hamlin RL, McCarthy PM, Bauer JA, Van Wagoner DR. Ascorbate attenuates atrial pacing-induced peroxynitrite formation and electrical remodeling and decreases the incidence of post-operative atrial fibrillation. *Circ. Res.* 2001;89:32−38.

[262] Vinay J, Rodrigo R. Postoperative atrial fibrillation. In: Rodrigo R, editor. Oxidative Stress and Antioxidants: Their role in Human Disease. New York, Nova Publishers. 2009. pp. 91-110.

[263] Korantzopoulos P, Kolettis TM, Kountouris E, Dimitroula V, Karanikis P, Pappa E, Siogas K, Goudevenos JA. Oral vitamin C administration reduces early recurrence rates after electrical cardioversion of persistent atrial fibrillation and attenuates associated inflammation. *Int. J. Cardiol.* 2005;102:321-326.

[264] Hicks JJ, Montes-Cortes DH, Cruz-Dominguez MP, Medina-Santillan R, Olivares-Corichi IM. Antioxidants decrease reperfusion induced arrhythmias in myocardial infarction with ST-elevation. *Front Biosci.* 2007;12:2029-2037.

[265] Eslami M, Badkoubeh RS, Mousavi M, Radmehr H, Salehi M, Tavakoli N, Avadi MR. Oral ascorbic acid in combination with beta-blockers is more effective than beta-blockers alone in the prevention of atrial fibrillation after coronary artery bypass grafting. *Tex. Heart Inst. J.* 2007;34:268-274.

[266] Castillo R. Metabolic Syndrome. In: Rodrigo R, editor. Oxidative Stress and Antioxidants: Their role in Human Disease. New York, Nova Publishers. 2009a. Pp. 159-192.

[267] Garcia-Diaz DF, Campion J, Milagro FI, Paternain L, Solomon A, Martinez JA. Ascorbic acid oral treatment modifies lipolytic response and behavioural activity but not glucocorticoid metabolism in cafeteria diet fed rats. *Acta Physiol.* (Oxf). 2008. Epub in Print.

[268] Hasegawa N, Niimi N, Odani F. Vitamin C is one of the lipolytic substances in green tea. *Phytother. Res.* 2002;16:S91–S92.

[269] Kodama M, Inoue F, Kodama T, Kodama M. Intraperitoneal administration of ascorbic acid delays the turnover of 3H-labelled cortisol in the plasma of an ODS rat, but not in the Wistar rat. Evidence in support of the cardinal role of vitamin C in the progression of glucocorticoid synthesis. *In Vivo.* 1996;10:97-102.

[270] Zhan CD, Sindhu RK, Vaziri ND. Up-regulation of kidney NAD(P)H oxidase and calcineurin in SHR: reversal by lifelong antioxidant supplementation. *Kidney Int.* 2004;65:219–227.

[271] Antoniades C, Tousoulis D, Tentolouris C, Toutouzas P, Stefanadis C. Oxidative stress, antioxidant vitamins, and atherosclerosis. From basic research to clinical practice. *Herz.* 2003;28:628–638.

[272] Abdel-Wahab Y, O'Harte F, Mooney M, Barnett C, Flatt P. Vitamin C supplementation decreases insulin glycation and improves glucose homeostasis in obese hyperglycemic (ob/ob) mice. *Metabolism.* 2002;51:514–517.

[273] Carcamo J, Pedraza A, Borquez-Ojeda O, Golde D. Vitamin C suppresses TNF alpha-induced NF kappa B activation by inhibiting I kappa B alpha phosphorylation. *Biochemistry.* 2002;41:12995–13002.

[274] Duarte TL, Lunec J. Review: when is an antioxidant not an antioxidant? A review of novel actions and reactions of vitamin C. *Free Radic. Res.* 2005;39:671–686.

[275] Houstis N, Rosen E, Lander E. Reactive oxygen species have a causal role in multiple forms of insulin resistance. 2006;440:944-948.

[276] Castillo R. Diabetes Mellitus. In: Rodrigo R, editor. Oxidative Stress and Antioxidants: Their role in Human Disease. New York, Nova Publishers. 2009b. pp. 193-222.

[277] Ceriello A, Lizzio S, Bortolotti N, Russo A, Motz E, Tonutti L, Crescentini A, Taboga C. Meal-generated oxidative stress in type 2 diabetic patients. *Diabetes Care.* 1998;21:1529-1533.

[278] Kuyvenhoven JP, Meinders AE. Oxidative stress and diabetes mellitus. Pathogenesis of long-term complications. *Eur. J. Intern. Med.* 1999;10:9-19.

[279] Kubisch HM, Wang J, Bray TM, Phillips JP. Targeted overexpression of Cu/Zn superoxide dismutase protects pancreatic beta-cells against oxidative stress. *Diabetes.* 1997;46:1563-1566.
[280] Xu B, Moritz JT, Epstein PN. Overexpression of catalase provides partial protection to transgenic mouse beta cells. *Free Radic. Biol. Med.* 1999;27:830-837.
[281] Hotta M, Tashiro F, Ikegami H, Niwa H, Ogihara T, Yodoi J, Miyazaki J.Pancreatic beta cell-specific expression of thioredoxin, an antioxidative and antiapoptotic protein, prevents autoimmune and streptozotocin-induced diabetes. *J. Exp. Med.* 1998;188:1445-1451.
[282] Chen H, Carlson EC, Pellet L, Moritz JT, Epstein PN. Overexpression of metallothionein in pancreatic beta-cells reduces streptozotocin-induced DNA damage and diabetes. *Diabetes.* 2001;50:2040-2046.
[283] Lenzen S, Drinkgern J, Tiedge M. Low antioxidant enzyme gene expression in pancreatic islets compared with various other mouse tissues. *Free Radic. Biol. Med.* 1996;20:463-466.
[284] Valko M, Leibfritz D, Moncol J, Cronin MT, Mazur M, Telser J. Free radicals and antioxidants in normal physiological functions and human disease. *Int. J. Biochem. Cell. Biol.* 2007;39:44-84.
[285] Lakey JR, Suarez-Pinzon WL, Strynadka K, Korbutt GS, Rajotte RV, Mabley JG, Szabó C, Rabinovitch A. Peroxynitrite is a mediator of cytokine-induced destruction of human pancreatic islet beta cells. *Lab. Invest.* 2001;81:1683-1692.
[286] Rabinovitch A, Suarez-Pinzon WL. Cytokines and their roles in pancreatic islet beta-cell destruction and insulin-dependent diabetes mellitus. *Biochem. Pharmacol.* 1998;55:1139-1149.
[287] Mabley JG, Rabinovitch A, Suarez-Pinzon W, Haskó G, Pacher P, Power R, Southan G, Salzman A, Szabó C. Inosine protects against the development of diabetes in multiple-low-dose streptozotocin and nonobese diabetic mouse models of type 1 diabetes. *Mol. Med.* 2003;9:96-104.
[288] Song Y, Song Z, Zhang L, McClain CJ, Kang YJ, Cai L. Diabetes enhances ipopolysaccharide-induced cardiac toxicity in the mouse model. *Cardiovasc. Toxicol.* 2003;3:363-372.
[289] Szabó C, Mabley JG, Moeller SM, Shimanovich R, Pacher P, Virag L, Soriano FG, Van Duzer JH, Williams W, Salzman AL, Groves JT. Part I: pathogenetic role of peroxynitrite in the development of diabetes and diabetic vascular complications: studies with FP15, a novel potent peroxynitrite decomposition catalyst. *Mol. Med.* 2002;8:571-580.

[290] Cameron NE, Cotter MA. Effects of antioxidants on nerve and vascular dysfunction in experimental diabetes. *Diabetes Res. Clin. Pract.* 1999;45:137-146.

[291] Rupérez FJ, García-Martínez D, Baena B, Maeso N, Cifuentes A, Barbas C, Herrera E. Evolution of oxidative stress parameters and response to oral vitamins E and C in streptozotocin-induced diabetic rats. *J. Pharm. Pharmacol.* 2008;60:871-878.

[292] Lee EY, Lee MY, Hong SW, Chung CH, Hong SY. Blockade of oxidative stress by vitamin C ameliorates albuminuria and renal sclerosis in experimental diabetic rats. *Yonsei Med. J.* 2007;48:847-855.

[293] Ajay M, Mustafa MR. Effects of ascorbic acid on impaired vascular reactivity in aortas isolated from age-matched hypertensive and diabetic rats. *Vascul. Pharmacol.* 2006;45:127-133.

[294] Baker TA, Milstien S, Katusic ZS. Effect of vitamin C on the availability of tetrahydrobiopterin in human endothelial cells. *J. Cardiovasc. Pharmacol.* 2001;37:333-338.

[295] Gormaz J, Rodrigo R. Nonalcoholic Steatohepatitis. In: Rodrigo R, editor. Oxidative Stress and Antioxidants: Their role in Human Disease. New York, Nova Publishers. 2009. pp- 223-256.

[296] Sokol RJ, McKim JM Jr, Goff MC, Ruyle SZ, Devereaux MW, Han D, Packer L, Everson G. Vitamin E reduces oxidant injury to mitochondria and the hepatotoxicity of taurochenodeoxycholic acid in the rat. *Gastroenterology.* 1998;114:164–174.

[297] Lenton KJ, Sané AT, Therriault H, Cantin AM, Payette H, Wagner JR.Vitamin C augments lymphocyte glutathione in subjects with ascorbate deficiency. *Am. J. Clin. Nutr.* 2003;77:189-195.

[298] Shireen KF, Pace RD, Mahboob M, Khan AT. Effects of dietary vitamin E, C and soybean oil supplementation on antioxidant enzyme activities in liver and muscles of rats. *Food Chem. Toxicol.* 2008;46:3290-3294.

[299] Kadirvel R, Sundaram K, Mani S, Samuel S, Elango N, Panneerselvam C. Supplementation of ascorbic acid and alpha-tocopherol prevents arsenic-induced protein oxidation and DNA damage induced by arsenic in rats. *Hum. Exp. Toxicol.* 2007;26:939-946.

[300] Halliwell B, Gutteridge JM. Free radicals in biology and Medicine. Oxford, Oxford University Press. 1999.

[301] Maxwell SR, Lip GY. Reperfusion injury: a review of the pathophysiology, clinical manifestations and therapeutic options. *Int. J. Cardiol.* 1997;58:95–117.

[302] Dhalla NS, Temsah RM, Netticadan T. Role of oxidative stress in cardiovascular diseases. *J. Hypertens.* 2000;18:655–673.

[303] Fliss H, Gattinger D. Apoptosis in ischemic and reperfused rat myocardium. *Circ. Res.* 1996;79:949–956.

[304] Granger DN. Role of xanthine oxidase and granulocytes in ischemia-reperfusion injury. *Am. J. Physiol.* 1988;255:1269–1275.

[305] Kang SM, Lim S, Song H, Chang W, Lee S, Bae SM, Chung JH, Lee H, Kim HG, Yoon DH, Kim TW, Jang Y, Sung JM, Chung NS, Hwang KC. Allopurinol modulates reactive oxygen species generation and Ca2+ overload in ischemia-reperfused heart and hypoxia-reoxygenated cardiomyocytes. *Eur. J. Pharmacol.* 2006;535:212–219.

[306] Tan S, Yokoyama Y, Dickens E, Cash T.G, Freeman B.A, Parks D.A. Xanthine-oxidase activity in the circulation of rats following hemorrhagic shock. *Free Radic. Biol. Med.* 1993;15:407–414.

[307] Terada LS, Dormish JJ, Shanley PF, Leff JA, Anderson BO, Repine JE. Circulating xanthine oxidase mediates lung neutrophil sequestration after intestinal ischemia-reperfusion. *Am. J. Physiol.* 1992;263:L394–L401.

[308] Grisham MB, Hernandez LA, Granger DN. Xanthine oxidase and neutrophil infiltration in intestinal ischemia. *Am. J. Physiol.* 1986;251:G567–G574.

[309] Zimmerman JJ. Defining the role of oxyradicals in the pathogenesis of sepsis. *Crit. Care Med.* 1995;23:616–617.

[310] Nathan AT, Singer M. The oxygen trail: tissue oxygenation. *Br. Med. Bull.* 1999;55:96–108.

[311] Macdonald J, Galley H.F, Webster N.R. Oxidative stress and gene expression in sepsis. *Br. J. Anaesth.* 2003;90 221–232.

[312] Petrich ER, Schanne OF, Zumino AP. Electrophysilogical responses to ischemia and reperfusion. In: Karmazyn M, ed.. Myocardial ischemia: mechanism, reperfusion, protection. *Basel, Birkhauser Verlag.* 1996. pp. 115–133.

[313] Kumar HS, Anandan R. Biochemical studies on the cardioprotective effect of glutamine on tissue antioxidant defense system in isoprenaline-induced myocardial infarction in rats. *J. Clin. Biochem. Nutr.* 2007;40:49–55.

[314] Lefer DJ, Granger DN. Oxidative stress and cardiac disease. *Am. J. Med.* 2000;109:315– 323.

[315] Duranteau J, Chandel NS, Kulisz A, Shao Z, Schumacker PT. Intracellular signaling by reactive oxygen species during hypoxia in cardiomyocytes. *J. Biol. Chem.* 1998;273:11619– 11624.

[316] von Harsdorf R, Li PF, Dietz R. Signaling pathways in reactive oxygen species-induced cardiomyocyte apoptosis. *Circulation.* 1999;99:2934–2941.

[317] Hensley K, Robinson KA, Gabbita SP, Salsman S, Floyd RA. Reactive oxygen species, cell signaling, and cell injury. *Free Radic. Biol. Med.* 2000;28:1456– 1462.

[318] Jaxa-Chamiec T, Bednarz B, Drozdowska D, Gessek J, Gniot J, Janik K, Kawka-Urbanek T, Maciejewski P, Ogórek M, Szpajer M. MIVIT Trial Group. Antioxidant effects of combined vitamins C and E in acute myocardial infarction. The randomized, double-blind, placebo controlled, multicenter pilot Myocardial Infarction and VITamins (MIVIT) trial. *Kardiol. Pol.* 2005;62:344-50.

[319] Jaxa-Chamiec T, Bednarz B, Herbaczynska-Cedro K, Maciejewski P, Ceremuzynski L. MIVIT Trial Group. Effects of vitamins C and E on the outcome after acute myocardial infarction in diabetics: a retrospective, hypothesis-generating analysis from the MIVIT study. *Cardiology.* 2009;112:219-223.

[320] Singh RB, Niaz MA, Rastogi SS, Rastogi S. Usefulness of antioxidant vitamins in suspected acute myocardial infarction (The Indian Experiment of Infarct Survival-3). *Am. J. Cardiol.* 1996;77:232-236.

[321] Laskowski H, Minczykowski A, Wysocki H. Mortality and clinical course of patients with acute myocardial infarction treated with streptokinase and antioxidants: mannitol and ascorbic acid. *Int. J. Cardiol.* 1995;48:235-237.

[322] Guaiquil V, Golde D, Beckles D, Mascareno E, Siddiqui M. Vitamin C inhibits hypoxia-induced damage and apoptotic signaling pathways in cardiomyocytes and ischemic hearts. *Free Radic Biol. Med.* 2004;37:1419–1429,

[323] Rohrbach S, Martin A, Niemann B, Cherubini A. Enhanced myocardial vitamin C accumulation in left ventricular hypertrophy in rats is not attenuated with transition to heart failure. *Eur. J. Heart Fail.* 2008;10:226-232.

[324] Rajan DP, Huang W, Dutta B, Devoe LD, Leibach FH, Ganapathy V, Prasad PD. Human placental sodium-dependent vitamin C transporter (SVCT2): molecular cloning and transport function. *Biochem. Biophys. Res. Commun.* 1999;262:762–768.

[325] Ribeiro DA, Buttros JB, Oshima CT, Bergamaschi CT, Campos RR. Ascorbic acid prevents acute myocardial infarction induced by isoproterenol in rats: role of inducible nitric oxide synthase production. *J. Mol. Histol.* 2009;40:99-105.

[326] Flamm, E. S, Demopoulos, H. B, Seligman, M. L, Poser, R. G, Ransohoff, J. Free radicals in cerebral ischemia. *Stroke.* 1978;9:445–447.

[327] Rehncrona S, Folbergrova J, Smith DS, Siesjo BK. Influence of complete and pronounced incomplete cerebral ischemia and subsequent recirculation on cortical concentrations of oxidized and reduced glutathione in the rat. *J. Neurochem.* 1980;34:477–486.

[328] Rice ME, Lee EJ, Choy Y. High levels of ascorbic acid, not glutathione, in the CNS of anoxia-tolerant reptiles contrasted with levels in anoxia-intolerant species. *J. Neurochem.* 1995;64:1790–1799.

[329] Ranjan A, Theodore D, Haran RP, Chandy MJ. Ascorbic acid and focal cerebral ischaemia in a primate model. *Acta Neurochir.* (Wien) 1993;123:87–91.

[330] Berger UV, Lu XC, Liu W, Tang Z, Slusher BS, Hediger MA. Effect of middle cerebral artery occlusion on mRNA expression for the sodium-coupled vitamin C transporter SVCT2 in rat brain. *J. Neurochem.* 2003;86:896–906.

[331] Huang J, Agus DB, Winfree CJ, Kiss S, Mack WJ, McTaggart RA, Choudhri TF, Kim LJ, Mocco J, Pinsky DJ, Fox WD, Israel RJ, Boyd TA, Golde DW, Connolly ES Jr. Dehydroascorbic acid, a blood–brain barrier transportable form of vitamin C, mediates potent cerebroprotection in experimental stroke. *Proc. Natl. Acad. Sci. U.S.A.* 2001;98:11720–11724.

[332] Mack WJ, Mocco J, Ducruet AF, Laufer I, King RG, Zhang Y, Guo W, Pinsky DJ, Connolly ES Jr. A cerebroprotective dose of intravenous citrate/sorbitol-stabilized dehydroascorbic acid is correlated with increased cerebral ascorbic acid and inhibited lipid peroxidation after murine reperfused stroke. *Neurosurgery.* 2006;59:383–388.

[333] González MJ, Miranda-Massari JR, Mora EM, Guzman A, Riordan NH, Riordan HD, Casciari JJ, Jackson JA, Roman-Franco A. Orthomolecular oncology review: ascorbic acid and cancer 25 years later. *Integr. Cancer.* Ther. 2005;4:32-44.

[334] Wang X, Liu J, Yokoi I, Kohno M, Mori A. Direct detection of circulating free radicals in the rat using electron spin resonance spectrometry. *Free Radic. Biol. Med.* 1992;12:121-6.

[335] Spellberg Ma, Keeton RW. Excretion of ascorbic acid in relation to saturation and utilization with some diagnostic implications. *Arch. Int. Med.* 1939;63:1095-1116.

[336] Bodansky O, Wroblewski F, Markardi B. Concentrations of ascorbic acid in plasma and white blood cells of patients with cancer and noncancerous chronic disease. *Cancer.* 1952;5:678-684.

[337] Holmes HN, Alexander W. Hay Fever and Vitamin C. *Science.* 1942;96:497-499.

[338] Holmes HN, Campbell K. The Determination of Vitamin C in Urine. *J. Lab. Clin. Med.* 1939;24:1293-1296.

[339] González MJ, Miranda-Massari JR, Mora EM, Jiménez IZ, Matos MI, Riordan HD, Casciari JJ, Riordan NH, Rodríguez M, Guzmán A. Orthomolecular oncology: a mechanistic view of intravenous ascorbate's chemotherapeutic activity. *P. R. Health Sci. J.* 2002;21:39-41.

[340] Cathcart RF. Vitamin C – the non-toxic, nonrated-limited, antioxidant free radical scavenger. *Med. Hypotheses.* 1985;18:61-77.

[341] Casciari J, Riordan N, Schmidt T, Meng X, Jackson JA, Riordan H. Cytotoxicity of ascorbate, lipoic acid and other antioxidants in hollow fiber in vitro tumors. *Br. J. Cancer.* 2001;84:1544-1550.

[342] Padayatty SJ, Levine M. Revaluation of ascorbate in cancer treatment: emerging evidence, open minds and serendipity. *J. Am. Coll. Nutr.* 2000;19:423-425.

[343] Leung PY, Miyashita K, Young M, Tsao CS. Cytotoxic effect of ascorbate and its derivatives on cultured malignant and nonmalignant cell lines. *Anticancer Res.* 1993;13:475-480.

[344] Sakagami H, Satoh K, Hakeda Y, Kumegawa M. Apoptosis-inducing activity of vitamin C and vitamin K. *Cell Mol. Biol.* (Noisy-le-grand). 2000;46:129-143.

[345] Riordan NH, Riordan HD, Casciari JP. Clinical and experimental experiences with intravenous vitamin C. *J. Orthomol. Med.* 2000;15:201-213.

[346] McCormick WJ. Cancer: a collagen disease, secondary to a nutritional deficiency. *Arch Pediatr.* 1959;76:166-171.

[347] Cameron E, Campbell A. The orthomolecular treatment of cancer. II. Clinical trial of high-dose ascorbic acid supplements in advanced human cancer. *Chem. Biol. Interact.* 1974;9:285-315.

[348] Cameron E, Pauling L. Supplemental ascorbate in the supportive treatment of cancer: reevaluation of prolongation of survival times in

terminal human cancer. *Proc. Natl. Acad. Sci. U. S. A.* 1978;75:4538-4542.

[349] Creagan ET, Moertel CG, O'Fallon JR, Schutt AJ, O'Connell MJ, Rubin J, Frytak S. Failure of high-dose vitamin C (ascorbic acid) therapy to benefit patients with advanced cancer. A controlled trial. *N. Engl. J. Med.* 1979;301:687-690.

[350] Moertel CG, Fleming TR, Creagan ET, Rubin J, O'Connell MJ, Ames MM. High-dose vitamin C versus placebo in the treatment of patients with advanced cancer who have had no prior chemotherapy. A randomized doubleblind comparison. *N. Engl. J. Med.* 1985;312:137-141.

[351] Wittes RE. Vitamin C and cancer [Editorial]. *N. Engl. J. Med.* 1985;312:178-179.

[352] Fairfield KM, Fletcher RH. Vitamins for chronic disease prevention in adults: scientific review. *JAMA*. 2002;287:3116-3126.

[353] Traipe L, Castillo R, Rodrigo R. Glaucoma. In: Rodrigo R, editor. Oxidative Stress and Antioxidants: Their role in Human Disease. New York, Nova Publishers. 2009. pp. 297-321.

[354] Wilkinson I, Megson I, MacCallum H. Oral vitamin C reduces arterial stiffness and platelet aggregation in humans. *J. Cardiovasc. Pharmacol.* 1999;34:690–693.

[355] Muller A, Pietri S, Villain M, Frejaville C, Bonne C, Culcas M Free radicals in rabbit retina under ocular hyperpressure and functional consequences. *Exp. Eye Res.* 1997;64:637-643.

[356] DiMattio J. Active transport of ascorbic acid into lens epithelium of the rat. *Exp. Eye Res.* 1989;49:873-885.

[357] Elmore AR. Final report of the safety assessment of L-Ascorbic Acid, Calcium Ascorbate, Magnesium Ascorbate, Magnesium Ascorbyl Phosphate, Sodium Ascorbate, and Sodium Ascorbyl Phosphate as used in cosmetics. *Int. J. Toxicol.* 2005;24:51-111.

[358] Evans J. Antioxidant supplements to prevent or slow down the progression of AMD: a systematic review and meta-analysis. *Eye.* 2008;22:751–760.

[359] Evans JR, Henshaw K. Antioxidant vitamin and mineral supplements for preventing age-related macular degeneration. *Cochrane Database Syst. Rev.* 2008;1: CD000253.

[360] Morris CD, Carson S. Routine vitamin supplementation to prevent cardiovascular disease: a summary of the evidence for the U.S. Preventive Services Task Force. *Ann. Intern. Med.* 2003;139:56–70.

[361] Frishman WH, Sinatra ST, Kruger N. Nutriceuticals and cardiovascular illness. In: Frishman WH, Weintraub MI, Micozzi M Eds.. Complementary and integrative therapies for cardiovascular disease. St Louis, MO, Elsevier. 2005. pp. 58–85.

[362] Kubler W, Gehler J. On the kinetics of the intestinal absorption of ascorbic acid: a contribution to the calculation of an absorption process that is not proportional to the dose. *Int. J. Vitam. Nutr. Res.* 1970;40:442–453.

[363] Schmidt KH, Hagmaier V, Hornig DH, Vuilleumier JP, Rutishauser G. Urinary oxalate excretion after large intakes of ascorbic acid in man. *Am. J. Clin. Nutr.* 1981;34:305–311.

[364] Urivetzky M, Kessaris D, Smith AD. Ascorbic acid overdosing: a risk factor for calcium oxalate nephrolithiasis. *J. Urol.* 1992;147:1215–1218.

[365] Massey LK, Liebman M, Kynast-Gales SA- Ascorbate increases human oxaluria and kidney stone risk. *J. Nutr.* 2005;135:1673–1677.

[366] Nankivell BJ, Murali KM. Images in clinical medicine. Renal failure from vitamin C after transplantation. *N. Engl. J. Med.* 2008;358: e4.

[367] McAllister CJ, Scowden EB, Dewberry FL, Richman A. Renal failure secondary to massive infusion of vitamin C. *JAMA.* 1984;252: 1684.

[368] Wong K, Thomson C, Bailey RR, McDiarmid S, Gardner J. Acute oxalate nephropathy after a massive intravenous dose of vitamin C. *Aust. N. Z. J. Med.* 1994;24:410–411.

[369] Mehta JB, Singhal SB, Mehta BC. Ascorbic acid induced haemolysis in G-6-PD deficiency. *Lancet.* 1990;336:944.

[370] Iwamoto N, Kawaguchi T, Horikawa K, Nagakura S, Hidaka M, Kagimoto T, Takatsuki K, Nakakuma H. Haemolysis induced by ascorbic acid in paroxysmal nocturnal haemoglobinuria. *Lancet.* 1994;343:357.

[371] Langlois MR, Delanghe JR, De Buyzere ML, Bernard DR, Ouyang J. Effect of haptoglobin on the metabolism of vitamin C. *Am. J. Clin. Nutr.* 1997;66:606–610.

[372] Bailey DM, Raman S, McEneny J, Young IS, Parham KL, Hullin DA, Davies B, McKeeman G, McCord JM, Lewis MH. Vitamin C prophylaxis promotes oxidative lipid damage during surgical ischemia–reperfusion. *Free Radic. Biol. Med.* 2006;40:591–600.

[373] Patterson JW. The diabetogenic effect of dehydroascorbic and dehydroisoascorbic acids. *J. Biol. Chem.* 1950;183:81–88.

[374] Hathcock JN, Azzi A, Blumberg J, Bray T, Dickinson A, Frei B, Jialal I, Johnston CS, Kelly FJ, Kraemer K, Packer L, Parthasarathy S, Sies H,

Traber MG. Vitamins E and C are safe across a broad range of intakes. *Am. J. Clin. Nutr.* 2005;81 736–745.

Index

A

B

C

F

G

H

I

J

K

L

M

N

O

P

Q

R